WOUNDED WARRIORS

The true story of a soldier in Vietnam, the emotional wounds inflicted and the incredible journey of self-discovery.

By

COLIN P SISSON

Total Press

Whangarei, New Zealand

TOTAL PRESS First edition printed 1993

TOTAL PRESS Second edition 2021

If there are any discrepancies, the Author and Publisher would like to be made aware of them and corrections will be made in future editions. It is believed that all acknowledgements and permissions for researched material have been obtained. If there are any inadvertent omissions in the acknowledgements will be pleased to make the necessary corrections in future printings of this book.

Produced and printed in 2021 by JOP, Whangarei, New Zealand.
Cover design by Fran Lawrence at JOP.

ISBN 978-0-473-60274-1

All enquiries about obtaining further copies of this book, go to website: colinsisson.com

COVER: EKN/67/130NN; 5 platoon, B Company, 7th Battalion Royal Australian Regiment (7 RAR), Courtesy Australian War Memorial.

DEDICATION

I dedicate this book to every one of us that has the courage to rise above our past traumas and emotional pain. To eventually feel gratitude for all life's gifts and lessons that are generously placed before us to further our evolution, to grow and find love, happiness and inner freedom.

I further dedicate this work to every man and woman from any war that were under the orders to take other people's lives, especially those who fought in Vietnam – Ally or Communist. May we learn the vital lesson that there are no lasting solutions through conflict.

CONTENTS

Acknowledgements		1
Members of 6 Platoon, V2 Company		2
Foreword		5
1	Memories	11
2	SAS Adventure	17
3	SAS training and preparation for Vietnam	27
4	Vietnam	35
5	Long Green	43
6	Nui Dat	49
7	First action	55
8	The 'missing' helicopter	65
9	My night of terror	75
10	Kathryn	87
11	The Tet Offensive	97
12	Dust Off	107
13	The battle	115
14	Cordon and search	123
15	Ambushed	137
Photo section		147
16	The VC are human after all	165
17	Winners and losers	173
18	Countdown to going home	181
19	The soldier had to die	187
20	Malaysia	197
21	The green, green grass of home	209
22	A Russian adventure	213
23	The precious gem I stole from Russia	223
24	Returning to Vietnam	229
25	Final words	241
Postscript: The healing process of self-discovery		245
About the author		247
V2 Company nominal roll		248
More books written by Colin P. Sisson		253

ACKNOWLEDGEMENTS

The following Acknowledgements are not necessarily in order of importance, but in the time sequence they played in my life.

RITA HENDERSON: For giving my life back through your love and care. You and every wife of a veteran should be awarded the Victoria Cross for your bravery of marrying such wounded souls.

MICHAEL FREEDMAN: For the wisdom and teachings of the Qabalah, and for showing me to see beyond my limited self.

KATHRYN RICHARDSON: for sharing in a vital part of my life and your encouragement for me to feel my feelings and be released from the pain.

MARINA KITCHATOVA: the gem I stole from Russia who shared in my healing while I wrote the first edition of *Wounded Warriors*. Who also accompanied me back to Vietnam and witnessed a major part of my healing.

MAGDALENA JANICKA; My close spiritual companion since 2001. 'Madzia' co-founded Integrative Presence with me through our work. I am deeply grateful to the closeness between us we have formed over the years in our inner adventurous journey together.

CECIL POA and BARRY TOOHILL. Both members of V2 Company who helped with quotations and accuracy of events. Thanks Guys.

MEMBERS OF SIX PLATOON, V2 COMPANY

Rank	Name	Given Names	Casualties
Lt.	Wilson	John Gilbert Hamish (Platoon Commander)	
Sgt	Whitworth	John Russell (Platoon Sergeant)	
Cpl	Hunter	Paul Paora *	WIA
Cpl	Runga	Joseph Te Okoro *	
Cpl	Vautier	Walter Stephen *	
Cpl	Whitaker	Thomas Douglas * (*Section Commanders)	
Pte	Awatere	W.R.	KIA
(transfered to W Company prior to V Company leaving for Vietnam and later killed in action).			
Pte	Burgering	Colin Richard	
Pte	Cowie	(Andy) Andrew Panton	
Pte	Dargaville	(Dick) Richard	
Pte	Duggan	Brendan Vincent	
Pte	Framhiem	William Taerikimataki	
Pte	Gaunt	George	
Pte	Haua	Allen George David	WIA
Pte	Heremaia	Michael	
Pte	Hoani	(Joe) Joseph	
Pte	Hunter	Tuakau	WIA
LCpl	Kingi	David Karepa Pukeho	
Pte	Linley	John Herbert	
Pte	Matene	Hohipa	
Pte	Mathews	Rex Jan	
Pte	McGee	Joseph Edward	
Pte	McPhail	Daniel James	
Pte	Mitchell	(Mitch) Vian Christopher	
Pte	Nant	Raymond Hardy	
Pte	Neame	(Blue) Roy Henry	

Rank	Name	Given Names	Casualties
Pte	Paterson	(I.B.) Ian Bruce	
Pte	Peddie	Graham John	
LCpl	Perawiti	Patrick Puke	
Pte	Ratima	(Des) Desmond	WIA
Pte	Rawiri	David	
Pte	Sadlier	Harry	
Pte	Simmons	Brian Thomas	
Pte	Sisson	(Sas) Colin Purvis	
Pte	Taare	(BB) Whare Mira	
Pte	Tawhara	John Robert Sydney	WIA
Pte	Tauhinu	(Grease Gun) Jock	
Pte	Tautau	Barney Te Whanauapani	
Pte	Tocher	James Conway	

Thank you for sharing in one of the most important chapters in my life. I honour the courage you all demonstrated in what was believed to be in defense of our Country.

FOREWORD

The wounds of the body heal quickly, but wounds of the mind and the emotions can last a lifetime.

The writing of this book, the years of research and experience in my healing, allowed me a different viewpoint. When we change our point of view, our reality also changes. By fathoming our thoughts and feelings where the pain of deep wounds lay dormant, a new point of view is created, which can release the pain of the mind and heart. When we become emotional warriors and find the courage to face our painful memories that harbour our suppressed and locked away fears, the pain is released.

I dedicate this book to all the fallen heroes. Alcoholics, drug addicts, sexual abuse victims, anyone who has been emotionally hurt as well as all war veterans with PTSD (Post Traumatic Stress Disorder). I particularly honour those who climbed back through their emotional turmoil to find themselves to love again and find the joy of living.

War is not a natural behaviour. It is an extension of humanity's battle against itself and is the result of failed diplomacy, as well as a failed human morality. It leaves in its wake broken bodies, damaged minds and shattered lives. No one is made for war. A physically, mentally, and emotionally healthy person is simply too sensitive for that dreadful experience. When a person is emotionally damaged before such a traumatic event, which most people are in varying degrees, particularly from childhood, the effects only increase the damage proportionately. I was certainly damaged from an upbringing in a loving, yet dysfunctional family. My parents separated when I was seven, creating a family split. Not an unusual event in many people's lives, but most never fully realize the damage we received as children in such an upheaval.

From a young age, I had been stirred by four uncles, all who had fought in The Second World War, two with the 8th Army in Libya and Italy against the Germans, another in the New Zealand Navy, and one in New Guinea against the Japanese. My stepfather, Charley also fought in Libya, but he never spoke a word about it.

I grew up hearing their war stories, which were mostly about the humorous adventures they all got up to. What they did not talk about was the pain, fear; the rivers of blood clogging the desert floor or shot-away jungle and the scattered human parts after a firefight with modern high velocity weapons. Never did they speak about the sleepless nights or the terrifying and recurring nightmares when they did sleep. Nor the constant need for alcohol and justifying war stories of the past just to function and give meaning to their lives. How I admired them and was so proud to have had such relatives and envious of their noble deeds. And they were noble, even heroic, to have put themselves through such dreadful events.

My intention is to write an anti-war book, while honouring the men and women who, through their courage and commitment, put their lives on the line in defence of their countries – friend or foe. And, for an impressionable youngster urging his uncles on for ever more interesting stories, little did I know that one day I would discover for myself the truth about the downside of humanity's brutality against itself and one another. I think war is the stupidest of all human behaviour, but not the men and women who faced that terrible ordeal. We can despise war, and at the same time honour the men and women who took part, who gave so much of themselves for what they believed in, at the time, on either side: the desire to serve their country. In its purest sense, it really means selfless service in defence of other human beings at the potential loss of one's own life.

Perhaps this idea is outdated, but let us not lose sight of the incredible courage each soldier displayed in their worst moments and at the depth of their despair. True courage is found when we feel discouraged. When afraid and act or if needed, remain still is the true meaning of this inner strength. Only those who have felt their fear have truly felt their courage. This is what we can honour because we have all been at that place.

The idea to write *Wounded Warriors* started just before I left New Zealand on a world lecture tour of my work in 1992. Whilst packing up the house in readiness for my departure, I stumbled across my old Vietnam diaries, three little books that I had never read, still wrapped in an old brown paper bag tied with a piece of string. Not knowing what to do with them, I tossed them into the bottom of my suitcase to perhaps read on my travels. Whilst in England, just before I left for Moscow in June, I experienced an incredibly powerful healing session. During it, I got in touch with the memories and the horror of the worst days of the Tet offensive, twenty-four years earlier. Subsequently, a week later, I met in Moscow an ex-Soviet Russian soldier who had fought on the opposite side as an instructor for the Viet Cong during the Tet Offensive at the same time I was there. We discussed as friends that perhaps we might even have traded fire during those desperate days and who allowed me to help in his healing, which was equally healing for me.

Two months later, I arrived in Canberra, Australia, just in time to witness the opening of the National Memorial to the Australian Forces who served in Vietnam. I stood in the midst of the crowd at that memorial service and quietly wept as I felt all the inspiration, pain and despair of the millions of young men and women who fought in that terrible war. I immediately returned to where I was staying, opened my case and there, on the top of my clothes, to my surprise, was the brown paper bag with my Vietnam diaries. How it found its way to the top of my clothes from the bottom remains a mystery to this day. I immediately began to read and then started to write. I finished the first edition four months later.

I have often wondered why the Vietnam war, compared with other wars, mentally screwed up so many people who fought there. I think one reason is that there was no front line in Vietnam. When you entered the country during the war, even in an administration role, you were on a battlefield for the entire time. There was never any respite from the fear of a surprise mortar attack, sniper fire, or enemy ambush during those endless patrols for the combatants. Even in well-defended bases, the danger was always present.

Another reason was that the dreadful close proximity of meeting the enemy in jungle warfare made it more terrifying. One moment you were alone, and the next was the sudden unexpected appearance of a black-shirted VC (Viet Cong) often from only a few steps away, trying to kill you. The one who fired first, or more accurately, survived.

General movement through the Vietnamese jungle and most patrols were mainly conducted in single file with two lead scouts in front. Our lead scouts, or 'point man' as the Americans called them, carried the greatest risk and were true heroes. Because of their training, skill, and courage, almost every frontal contact we had, our scouts won the initial firefight. I was briefly a lead scout on one operation and knew how harrowing it was. Although sometimes the enemy bumped into us or ambushed us in the middle of our strung-out line or at our rear, meaning that there was no real safe place to be during a patrol.

Another terrifying aspect was the enemy snipers that took so many Allied lives throughout the war. Fortunately, V2 Company did not suffer any casualties from this threat, but the danger was always there. I had my own unfortunate and near fatal encounter with one.

Another chilling aspect was the constant threat of well-hidden enemy booby traps and, seeing your comrade right next to you, having his leg blown off from treading on one. Or stepping into the well hidden and dreaded punji pits full of sharpened bamboo spikes, smeared with human excrete. These caused dreadful wounds, and often a slow, lingering, and painful death. Who could ever say that war is glorious? Only those who had never experienced the blood, the horror, and the fear.

Another cause of pain for veterans, which most do not want to admit to, was that we actually lost the war that should never have been fought in the first place. That major factor that decided the outcome was because the enemy were fighting for their families, their wives and children, their country, even for their very lives. Their dedication was so great that despite being outnumbered, outgunned in firepower, outmaneuvered, and often outfought, they still won. Napoleon once said that 'morale is worth three times that of equipment'. The New Zealanders were among the few units that were completely made up of professional and highly motivated volunteers. This was reflected in the number of our losses in relation to the enemy killed, which was only one to every fifty-enemy, by body count. Yet, despite this military superiority, our purpose for being there could never rival that of the Vietnamese people's motivation to win. The eventual defeat of the South Vietnamese Government in 1975 caused most of us veterans some pain when we remembered fallen friends.

A further factor in the war that was so demoralising and dehumanizing to all those who were in combat was the lack of chivalry on the battlefield. Either side rarely honoured the life of the enemy. I remember hearing my uncles talk about the honour that was shared, with some exceptions, between the Germans and the Allies. Yet, there was still a lack of respect for human life, which is the main reason that keeps wars happening, and no more so than in Vietnam.

The success or failure of any mission was measured not by the amount of ground captured or held, or lives saved because of an engagement, but by the number of enemy killed in ratio to our own losses. This kill-rate factor epitomizes the stupidity and horror at the combat level. Markedly, this caused a moral drift of every individual taking part into deeper brutality, savagery, and the departure of their own humanness. This caused huge trauma in the young men and women on both sides of the conflict and took me over twenty years to start to recover from it.

Our homecoming was probably the biggest reason for the mental damage that New Zealand Vietnam veterans experienced. I remember the excitement I felt before arriving home, expecting a hero's welcome, perhaps a march down the main street in Auckland, accompanied by marching bands and waving crowds. But instead, having disembarked from the aircraft, lined up on the tarmac and to hear the following words from an administrative officer, the poor man being labelled angrily by several guys as a mere office clerk:

"Welcome home. After you are dismissed from this parade, get out of uniform, and tell no one where you have been. Dismiss!"

That's it? Is that all we are greeted with? The lack of acknowledgement of what we had been through in the defence of our nation was crushing. Acknowledgement from the New Zealand Government did gratefully come years later, but the psychological damage was already done.

Viewed historically, no one doubts that the war was a waste of time, resources, and a moral degradation of human decency, as all wars are. Not only for those who fought in it, but also for the entire world. I repeat, because of its importance. '*No lasting solution can ever be found through conflict.*' When will the world wake up to this?

Perhaps the only winners were the Vietnamese people who finally got their country back after being occupied by the French, the Japanese and the well-known corrupt South Vietnamese government that was supported by the Americans. They finally won peace, but at an appalling cost of millions killed and many millions more traumatized. I bow my head in deep respect and mourning for their pain.

For me personally, what was not a waste of time was the actual experience itself, for it opened parts of my subconscious that such a powerful event can often reach. And this is the story I want to tell, for it showed me that potentially, any highly traumatic event holds a blessing in the seed to an inner 'awakening.' War, as with any traumatic event, brings the worst and the best out in people. I was witness to both not only in others but also in myself. But what was more important to me was that it gave me a glimpse of myself at a deeper spiritual level that such an extreme situation can often give, and for that I am most grateful for.

This has not been the most enjoyable book I have ever written, but it has been the most powerful. I have tried to be as honest as I can while pulling no punches. It is frank, brutal, and softened with touches of humour. I trust it will get many who read it in touch with their own 'Inner Vietnam', their own fears and passions for living. I hope you are disgusted, amused and perhaps even inspired by this work as I was in writing it.

Each member of V2 had their own unique experience based upon their choices and reactions to what they were subjected to. Even though this is my story, it is essentially the story of every member of V Company, indeed every person who ever served in Vietnam, or in any war zone. It is probably the story of every person who ever faced appalling situations that led to being psychologically damaged. Each person, to some degree, has a suppressed battlefield inside of them and is a wounded warrior. It is my sincere hope that every veteran, and every person,who has experienced trauma, will one day be able to accept the past as a gift. This will signal a sure sign of their healing.

Thankyou
Colin P. Sisson
"Mo tetahi wā iti, me hikoi tahi tātou ki a tiria ngā whākaaro"
"Let us walk together for a while and share our thoughts."

1
MEMORIES

I lit a cigarette to do something with my hands and take my mind off what was stirring inside me. My therapist didn't mind me smoking, suggesting that it may help to relax me.

"What are you feeling, Colin?"

God, she was asking me to feel again. I looked at my feet to avoid her gaze, and her searching questions.

"Just relax Colin and know that you are safe right now."

Sure, I am safe right now, but how can I escape feelings I can't describe, or even feel properly? How can I get away from the memories of seeing men die and being part of that dreadful process? From the regular recurring nightmare of my own death with a bullet through the face. The memories of men with horrific wounds, screaming in the night, clogging my ears and mind with an endless scream of my own, but never daring to let it out. The smell of cordite from gunfire and exploding shells that clung to the air, filling my nostrils with its acrid odor. This smell had become synonymous with fear, horror, and terribly mutilated dead bodies. How could I speak or want to remember?

At last, I was relieved to hear her words signaling the end of the therapy session.

"Well, that will do for today. I'll see you again next week, Colin."

I nodded and slowly rose out of my chair. Smiling mechanically at her, I headed for the door, to be lost again in a world of normality that had no real meaning for me. A life of being a father, husband, salesman, student of business management, economics, and philosophy that I studied in my spare time. Philosophy was the only thing I could relate to, as it took me away from feelings that were ever ready to explode their violence and anger on to the rest of my life at the slightest provocation. Feelings that I wanted to escape from or forget.

This had been my sixth therapy session, with little to show for it. As much as I wanted to be free of what was going on inside me, I resisted looking within, much to the frustration of my therapist. I decided not to go back, and perhaps try something else.

It was 1979. Here I was, a father of two daughters who were the most precious things in the world to me, and yet emotionally I was unavailable to them. I knew this, but felt powerless to do anything about it.

Rita, my wife, had given me so much of herself throughout our marriage. We had met through the local Karate club, where I worked out most nights. I was physically fit, with an outgoing personality and a good sense of humour – wonderful disguises for a mind in torture, and unconsciously crying out to be loved.

It began on a blind date, soon after my return from Vietnam in 1969. She entered the room where I was waiting to meet her for the first time, by doing cartwheels across the floor, and ending up in a chair facing me. "Hi! I'm Rita." It was love at first sight with this amazing woman.

We dated regularly after that and felt we had both come home to each other. However, we both knew something was wrong with me early in our relationship.

One evening we were riding in a bus through the main street of Auckland and turned a corner. There, spread across the road, was an anti-Vietnam demonstration. I looked out at these people with a feeling of distaste and irritation. Then I saw a Communist North Vietnamese flag waving in the crowd as if beckoning me to react and react I did. Suddenly, I saw friends, Stuart Ellwood and Des Hirini, both killed in Vietnam, and the haggard, despairing look on young men's faces that had aged 10 years in a matter of days, from the constant exposure to combat. The fear and pain we had suffered that these protesters had no respect for caused an uncontrollable anger to well up in me.

I leapt up onto my seat backrest, with my face turned sideways, and through the open, narrow bus ventilation window, I shouted at the top of my voice every swear word my tongue could utter. I was beside myself with blind rage and in full combat mode. The driver stopped the bus and came running back to where I was now standing, on top of the back seat rest, screaming at the outside crowd. He glanced at Rita for an explanation and probably thought I was having an epileptic fit. Rita was wide-eyed with shock at what was happening to me.

"He's just returned from fighting in Vietnam, but I've never seen him like this," she said apologetically to the bus driver.

The driver gently touching my arm brought me back to reality.

"It's okay, son," he said, soothingly and with firm, caring hands, gently helped me down from my perch until I was back in my seat. "Are you all right now? You just sit there and relax," his comforting voice calmed my shaking body.

Rita put her arm around me as she wiped the spittle from my chin. "Thank you. I think he'll be alright now," she assured the driver.

I looked around, feeling disorientated and foolish. Everyone in the crowded bus was standing and staring at me with looks of concern on their faces. They all sat down, some shaking their heads in bewilderment, as the bus moved off. We got off at the next stop, before our destination, from embarrassment to stay on the bus.

Years later, I would agree with the protesters against the war. But then I took it personally and saw them despising us soldiers for having been there.

We were married early in 1971. I was 25 and Rita was 20, and neither of us was prepared for what lay ahead.

Our first child, Bernadette was born in late 1971, a little red-headed beauty with a spirit neither Rita nor I could handle. Bernadette was overly sensitive and quickly picked up on my fears and feelings of inadequacy. If she cried for any length of time, I became extremely anxious. She was weaned early but unbeknown to us, was allergic to cow's milk, and would cry for hours from desperation, pain, and hunger. I was beside myself during most of this time. We never sought help from the family because we were too proud to ask. Our repeated visits to the doctor were merely met with assurances that we were just overanxious and inexperienced parents. He was certainly right on both counts. We nearly lost Bernadette, and fortunately, the problem was picked by the Plunket (baby care) nurse who visited once a week. Though the situation improved after that, I was by that stage convinced I was a failure as a father.

Angela followed nearly two years later, but it was much easier because we were more experienced.

By 1973, nearly five years after my Vietnam tour, the recurring nightmare of me being shot in the face and burning to death from napalm bombs had almost stopped. Near the end of my tour while still in Vietnam, this dream happened every night, but it became less frequent as time passed. I thought that at last I had fully recovered from the whole grim experience. Rita gave me so much love and support through my pain, and would sit with me, holding my trembling body for hours during the night, as I was often too frightened to go back to sleep.

I began to study psychology at the local night university (technical institute) and read every book on the subject, along with books on philosophy that I could lay my hands on. Not only to help myself but also to explore the part of my mind that gave me a totally bizarre and weird experience while in Vietnam. It had happened three times and was during my worst moments in battle, when I was sure I was going to die. On one occasion when all hell was being released around me, with men screaming and dying, suddenly my whole reality changed, and everything began to move in seemingly slow motion. I found I had time to do several things quickly: dive for cover, return fire towards the enemy and change my empty rifle magazine. Then a feeling that I could only describe as a state of total bliss, in every part of my being, yet with no thoughts, no physical or mental stress, just a deep love greater than I had ever known.

Some of what I was reading called this an altered state of consciousness or an expanded state of awareness beyond or transcending experience. These explanations seemed too philosophical or mystical and only increased my confusion over what had happened to me. This further compounded when I remembered that whatever I could call it – 'love or bliss' (poor descriptions of what I had felt) extended to the enemy and I could no longer fire at my brothers in a different uniform. This incredible feeling differed from the delusional euphoric and closed or suppressed frozen state that many men experienced in combat as an automatic coping mechanism. It was different because I was completely carefree and fully present with everything that was happening outside and inside myself. I didn't know how long it lasted each time, but it soon passed and everything sped up to its normal speed again the second I thought about what was happening to me, along with the return of the fear and horror.

I often wondered about those experiences, and the part of the mind that caused such a thing to happen. Psychology did not answer this for me, but it gave me a wonderful platform for research of the fight/flight/freeze syndrome (the fear response) which later became the basis of my psychological work. But, back in 1979, I used my studies first to satisfy my curiosity, but then, as feelings from the war got stirred, to use my newfound psychological skills as just another way to avoid my suppressed feelings. I could be so wise and intellectual; a perfect disguise to hide my pain. This delayed my healing for many years.

About this time, I started as a student at the School of Philosophy. They fascinated me with their approach, which emphasized non-attachment, self-awareness, and the enslavement of the unconscious mechanical programmes of human thought, emotions, and behaviour. This, according to them, separated people from their latent powers of love, happiness, and inner freedom. That people relied on substitutes like drugs, alcohol, careers, and relationships instead of searching inside to where their actual power lay hidden.

One night after class, I casually asked the tutor what was the source of what we were studying. His reply was that it was not important for me to know. But then, I had to know, and spent the next two months combing the library shelves, trying to find what seemed to be unobtainable. Then one day, while visiting a friend, I found what I was looking for, in a book entitled, 'In search of the Miraculous', by P D Ouspensky. It described the work of George Gurdjieff, the Russian mystic who began teaching in Russia just before the first world war. He later moved his school to France, where it became famous for his unconventional approach to consciousness expansion.

For the next five years, I became a fanatical follower of Gurdjieff's teachings, which caused me to question all my old values. During this time, I also studied comparative religion, with an emphasis on Buddhism, Hindu philosophy, and a little Taoism. Then I discovered the Qabalah, and my most important spiritual teacher up to that time, Michael Freedman.

By now, my near total preoccupation with my personal philosophy and academic studies, along with my work, was causing our marriage to fall apart. A woman can only take so much of a man who simply was not 'there' emotionally as well as physically. It was years later before I realised my studies were just another avoidance of the pain locked up inside of me.

I continued to insist to myself that the war had not affected me and that if it had; I was now fully recovered. This idea came into some doubt when I was asked to give a talk on Vietnam to the local Historical Society one Sunday afternoon. I began to show the audience of about fifty people some coloured slides from my personal collection from the war. Within twenty minutes of my talk and after having shown half the slides, I was overcome with extreme feelings that ranged from anger to despair and probably was a panic attack. Unable to cope, I gathered up my slide projector and equipment and, without a further word, walked out on my startled audience. I walked through a park for three hours, fighting the tension in my body, and a cramping sense of loss so deep that I wanted to burst out crying. Yet I wouldn't let the tears come. After successfully suppressing all my emotions, I returned home and never said a word about the meeting to anyone.

Then in February 1980, I met John Wolfe, who was conducting a workshop on breathing, which he called Rebirthing. Initially, I was skeptical. But during the breathing session, I reconnected with the same altered state of consciousness I'd experienced in Vietnam that changes the passage of time to an instant – the full present moment. Not only that, but I also experienced the first few moments of my physical birth thirty-four years earlier and released the trauma of that painful event. I now understood why it was called 'Rebirthing.' This technique became the basis of my personal research from then on, and the inspiration for my future writing of books on the subject. Here at last was a process that got me out of my head, and back into my emotions and physical body in a safe and unobtrusive way. It was an event that was to change the course of my life.

I expanded on the breathing technique by adding processes I was learning from the Gurdjieff and Qabalah work. Thus changed the name from Rebirthing to Breath Integration, and years later in my work with Magdalena Janicka in Poland to Integrative Presence as we researched and expanded our understanding of the elusive present moment and expanded awareness. But then, I was only at the beginning and still had much healing before me from Vietnam.

Rita and I separated a few months later, and my world fell apart.

I was trying to hold down a job as a branch manager for a large chain of nursery furniture stores, while also studying at night university doing part-time counselling. It was probably the unhappiest time in my life. Deciding to give up all my counselling work, knowing I needed to work on myself for some time. With regular sessions from John, and then with a woman therapist, who started to open the unconscious and deeply suppressed parts of me, along with memories, my psychological wounds began to heal.

2

MY SAS ADVENTURE AND THE GRUELING SELECTION COURSE

I initially applied to join the famous Special Air Service (SAS) not because I ever planned to go to war, but from a youthful romantic zest for adventure. It was many years later that I fully realized my time with them saved me from the very worst traumatic effects of the war in preparing me through their meticulous training methods, and I am forever grateful for it.

The SAS adventure started in 1964 when I was 18 and thumbing through a local newspaper where I came across an advertisement 'A special kind of man. Join the elite unit of 1st Ranger Squadron of the New Zealand Special Air Service.'

That was it, and I was determined to join and be such a man. From that day, I started preparing myself in every way I could think of. My goal was to pass the gruelling ten-day selection course that only about 15% of participants ever pass. I gave myself a year to prepare, which included running 10 kilometres most days. During the rugby Union season, I played rugby every weekend. In addition, at the urging of my father, two nights a week I would run to rugby practice, which was 6 kilometres away, train for two hours and then run home again. Being physically underdeveloped from a sickly childhood, I regularly worked out with weights and muscle-building exercises. I even joined the local parachute club to see if I had the courage for it and completed nine jumps before signing up.

I was standing, lined up with 64 other hopefuls before the Squadron,

Sergeant Major Shaw, nicknamed 'shocker Shaw' because of his highly rigorous discipline and hard driving training methods. He had been in the British Commandos during the Second World War and had been on many commando raids against the Germans. He was a hard man that we were all going to discover soon enough. Coldly eyeing each of us, he bellowed out the rules of the coming ten days, and completed with:

"Know that you can drop out at any time and according to Major Mace, The Squadron's Commanding Officer, it will be no dishonour. But, to me, you look like a bunch of pussies. Less than 20 of you will be still standing at the end anyway, and that's only if you're lucky."

It was 1965. I was 19, one of the youngest and smallest in the squad, had the mental maturity of a 15-year-old and was still clinging to romantic and idealistic notions. I felt a little intimidated as I looked around at the others, more mature, some already with many years' military experience, bigger and I imagined more able to be the tough Special Forces soldier. But I had one advantage, and that I was super fit. My Father had said that if you are physically fit, you can put up with almost anything. He was only partly right as I learned from this coming 10 days and the following 3 years that there is a mental and emotional fitness that was far more important. It was here that we found our courage and inner strength. It was here that my success of passing the 10-day selection course or not would hang in the balance.

As part of my preparation for the SAS 10-day selection course, I devised a clever plan. Three months earlier, at the start of my basic army training, I had an extra thick sole put on a pair of boots, making them heavier. The idea was to get used to running for long distances with them to augment my fitness even more. I bought a second pair from the army store that was much lighter, which I planned to wear during the coming selection course, and I smiled at my thoughtfulness. But my clever plan lacked experience and was to seriously backfire on me. The 3 months basic had allowed me to slowly break in the heavier boots, moulding them to my feet. But, once the SAS selection course started in its intensity, there was no time to break in the lighter new boots. By the end of the second day, my feet ached from the new unadjusted boots, and by the fourth day, blisters appeared from the constant running. This was my worst mistake that I deeply regretted with every step. One of the more experienced participants showed me how to deal with blisters by putting a cotton thread through the blister with a needle, allowing the fluid to drain out, while keeping the skin to protect the wound. This helped for a while. I could not get my heavier, already broken-in boots, as I'd left them at my civilian address on my last leave. As the days rolled by, wearing such footwear became a torture that was a major test on its own.

The first day of the selection course wasn't so hard and the first part was mostly in being supplied and checking equipment. They issued us with a 303 rifle, a relic of the second world war that had ended only 20 years earlier.

Then the activities were divided up between extensive physical exertion (running long distance in full battle equipment) and mental short-term memory retention tests, with no breaks in between. This had the effect of exhausting us physically and mentally and then seeing how we would perform under such mental pressure. My physical fitness carried me well on this first day, and I felt I did okay.

The second day was harder, with longer runs and obstacles to run, climb and crawl over or under, with each activity running into the next. They did not give us any time to catch our breath or gather our thoughts that exhausted and drained our willpower. At the same time, they constantly harassed us with insults and drummed up punishments.

"What are you smiling at, soldier?" The sergeant would yell at the next victim, his face only centimetres away.

"I'm not smiling, sergeant!"

"Are you calling me a liar? On the ground and do 20 press ups, you piece of shit." They were doing their best to break us. 'I can keep doing this,' I determined to myself.

The next day was to test our leadership, problem solving and decision making.

We were put into groups of 5 and they selected one to be the team leader, who was given instructions for a task to be solved. Tasks ranged from having to change the wheel of a truck with no tools, to commanding a squad to rescue hostages from terrorists. Mine was solving a behind the line's scenario of one of my team becoming insane and threatening to shoot us, and giving our position away to the enemy. It played into my young, romantic idealism, and I felt I did well.

The rest of the day was along similar lines and I further felt confident that so far, I was doing okay, despite the increasing pain in my feet. But at 2 am the next morning, I began to lose my confidence. We were abruptly woken and ordered outside in full battle order and made to walk–run–walk for 15 kilometres along a bush track that led through a native forest. The worst part was that several times we had to wade up to our necks through freezing cold rivers and then continue the forced march in water-soaked equipment and clothes, adding extra kilos of weight, as well as huge discomfort. It was wintertime in New Zealand and the rivers were extremely cold. Often, we were confronted with tempting words, "You look tired, Sisson. Come on, you don't have to do this. There is a lovely hot breakfast and a warm bed waiting for you and a vehicle around the corner to take you home. You don't have to put up with this shit anymore."

After about 13 Kilometres and the third river, I was close to breaking. I asked the SAS sergeant if there were any more rivers to go through. I decided that, if so, I was going to quit. His response was, "Maybe, maybe not. You will have to see."

'Okay,' I said to myself, 'the next river, I will quit.' Two kilometres on with no more rivers, we came to our trucks that would take us back to camp. That had been the closest to quitting so far and felt it was a stroke of luck that I was still going.

Another disconcerting situation was sometimes during meals, we were suddenly interrupted halfway through with: "On your feet, outside and put on your equipment for a 10-kilometre run. Hey, you," pointing to some person who was slow to move.

"Leave that food alone and get outside if you don't want to feel the sole of my boot up where it hurts the most. Get moving!"

Some guys who had been at the back of the meal line barely had two mouthfuls before the interruption, and those at the front had to run on a full stomach, occasionally causing them severe stomach upset and one even to vomit. This happened three times during the course. When someone complained about how digestively unhealthy and upsetting this was, the answer was always the same: "If you are behind enemy lines, you will be lucky to find time, even to eat at all. Get moving, you useless son of a shit."

Each day blurred into a stream of unbelievable discomfort and pain as guys fell out and returned to their units. By day 5, we were down to 30, less than half from the starting group.

On day six at midday, they briefed us for the coming three days for an exercise called escape and evasion. "You are behind enemy lines" (yet again) "and the local population is hostile, so avoid them at all times. You have three days to get from point A to point B. I suggest you travel at night to avoid getting caught. Each will be given a map, compass, and a grid reference where you must get to where friendly forces will pick you up. I suggest you commit to memory the map grid reference of your RV (rendezvous) and then destroy it. If you are caught with the grid reference, or you divulge it if captured, many friendly people will be arrested and executed. That is the scenario. Later this afternoon, you will be driven to your starting point and individually dropped off. Don't team up with any other participant, so you must stay alone. You have three days to travel forty kilometres over steep hills, farmland, swamps, thick bush, and forest to reach your RV. During this time a unit of infantry, elements of the police and SAS troops will search to capture you. If you are caught, we will severely interrogate you for the location of your RV."

"What will you do to us if we are caught and not tell you our RV location?" one asked. Shocker Shaw's reply was:

"You don't want to know. It will make all the discomfort you have experienced so far, like a walk in the park. We have interrogation officers who are specially trained, and I can tell you, they WILL get that information from you. So, do not get caught. Any other questions before we have a quick break?"

During the break, one of our group started saying.

"I heard about one participant from the last selection course, who got caught on this escape and evasion exercise. They made him kneel on a wire fence with his full weight and gear until he talked."

"They can't do that. We are not real enemies," another chimed in.

"Well, what they have done to us so far, I wouldn't be surprised at what they might do. Anyway, I don't know if it is true or not, but let me tell you, I am sure as hell not going to get caught." We all nodded our full agreement.

They provided us with only one day's rations for the coming three days. As our truck drove through the late afternoon with drizzling rain, I was already distributing in my mind my meagre food supply to ensure that I will eat something no matter how little every 4 hours to keep myself going.

These three days were a blessing and a break from the constant harassment, sleep and meal interruptions, the forced marches, and exercises. For three days I could go at my own pace, even if I am a little hungry. I would travel at night and catch up on sleep during the day, as they suggested. I studied my map, having already memorized the RV map grid reference, and destroyed the written evidence. I was excited, confident, and it all seemed like an adventure, even a game. As long as I reached the RV in time, points were lost if we were late or early, and each participant had to arrive at their set hour, within a half an hour variation, to not all arrive at the same time. It impressed me how well they had planned it out.

Finally, my turn came to leap from the slow-moving truck and made my way into the tree line off the road. There was a beach and a coastal road that led directly to the rendezvous forty kilometres away, but they had warned us that both would be heavily patrolled and to stay off them. 'Move inland, even though the going would be harder, there would be fewer patrols and more cover,' they had advised. I moved inland in dense bush and waited for dark. Had a small meal and then started.

It seemed impossible! I had barely covered 100 metres in an hour. The bush was so thick, and it was so dark. At this rate, it would take me a week to arrive. Two hours later, with no better terrain and becoming exhausted, I decided to move towards the coastal road and reasoned that if I was extra careful, I could catch up a lot of lost time. Three hours later, I arrived and after watching for any 'enemy' movements, I slowly and carefully made my way along the deserted road. It seemed like it was a good decision because in 30 minutes I had covered a whole kilometre, saving time and energy, and smiled to myself.

Suddenly, from 20 metres away, a set of headlights came to life and caught me in its glare. I heard a voice saying, "There's one, get him." With doors opening, closing, boots hitting the road and the engine of the land rover bursting into life, reeved in my direction. I panicked as my worst fears had happened. I sprinted down the road pursued by three running sets of boots and a speeding land rover. I saw a small clearing to my left leading into the bush and sprinted into it. Knowing my pack was slowing me down, I ripped it off my back and, with my cumbersome webbing, threw them into a small bush and, with a new lightness with just my rifle, sprinted down a bush track. The pursuers, as well as the land rover had seen me move down the bush road, turned to follow me. Around a corner where I was no longer in the headlights' glare, I dived into a bush and waited, daring not to breathe as I heard the approaching troopers. I was truly terrified as it was no longer a game as the prospect of being caught was upon me.

"Where did he go?" One muttered, as he shone a torch into the bush only a metre away from where I was lying. I froze, knowing that the slightest movement would give me away. They all went past, not seeing me.

10 Minutes later they returned, but now more carefully checking each side of the bush track with torches. Meantime, I had moved a few metres deeper into the bush, then remained perfectly still. They passed, and all was quiet for the next 20 minutes I lay there for, before daring to move. Then, quietly moved back along the track and spent over an hour searching

for my gear. I was about to give up, concluding that they had found it, when relieved to find it with my precious little food, a change of clothes, sleeping bag and lightweight shelter. Checking my compass, I made my way inland and would venture nowhere near the coast with a lesson well learnt. It was hard going and by 4 am, totally exhausted, I had finally reached open farmland and cleared the bush with much relief.

Within half an hour, I found a farmer's barn and carefully opened the barn door with a loud creaking sound and saw it was full of hay bales. 'Oh, heaven,' and climbing a ladder up to an upstairs loft, and crawling into the dry space, I changed out of my wet clothes, had a mouthful of nuts and, in my sleeping bag, was asleep within seconds.

I woke at midday, and it had stopped raining but was still threatening with more to come. As I peeked out to my surroundings, I was delighted to find a field of turnips nearby, after ensuring no one was about, I crept to the edge of the turnip field and with my bayonet dug up one of the precious vegetables, pearled of the dirt and skin and dropped the raw piece into my mouth. It was the best tasting turnip I ever had. I dug up 4 more large turnips and retreated to my barn just as it started to rain again, to enjoy a good meal. Climbing back into my sleeping bag, I dozed for a few hours.

I was suddenly jolted awake with the creaking of the barn door opening, causing me to freeze. Hearing some movement below, I carefully peeked to see a farmer and a dog below me on the barn floor. The dog instantly saw me and started barking. I hid myself, hoping it would stop, but it didn't. The farmer scolded the animal.

"Shut up you stupid mutt, it's only a rat. Come on, let's go." Again, I had the barn to myself.

After a small meal, I changed back into my cold, wet clothes, and it was such a torture, but it ensured that I would always have dry clothes to sleep in. One of the SAS lectures had been strict about this, and a year later, on an SAS training exercise, a trooper failed to observe this and died from hypothermia.

Shivering in the wet clothes, I left my refuge and set off. It was at 6 pm and was just getting dark, so headed towards the tree line and continued moving through the bush for the next 10 hours. I had lost a lot of time and needed to catch up, stopping to rest and eat something every hour and to ease the pain of my blistered feet. That was really slowing me down, but I was determined to keep going.

The rest of the trip was uneventful and made it to the RV with 25 minutes to spare. That night back at the barracks, we all shared our stories. There were many amazing adventures that brought lots of laughs and relief that we had only one day to go. The best story was one guy on the first night came to a small cottage and saw through the window an attractive young woman. After ensuring she was alone, knocked on the door to ask for a cup of sugar.

"Bloody hell, you could have thought up something more original than that." Cut in one of his listeners.

"Well, it seems to have worked because she invited me in for a cup of tea. That led to being invited for a meal, a bed and, yes, you guessed it. We spent the next 3 days in glorious lovemaking, eating, drinking and a half an hour before my meeting, she ran me in her car and dropped me off just short of the RV."

"That's cheating," one chipped in.

"Well, they told us to use our ingenuity." He replied. Another chimed in, "If I am ever stuck behind enemy lines, I will make sure that I am with you." We all laughed.

That night, they let us eat and sleep uninterrupted, which made us all uneasy about what they had in store for us on the last day. At 7 am only 16 of us were left and we all nervously stood on parade, standing at attention in the cold drizzling rain waiting for Shocker Shaw to appear. We had been right to have been nervous. His opening words when he appeared 10 minutes late (on purpose) with us all shivering with the cold wet, were:

"Okay, you bastards, fetch your equipment and in ten minutes we leave for a 20-kilometre run in full battle gear. You will have breakfast when we get back. Move!"

This was my worst nightmare. I knew my feet would not stand this final torture of the longest run so far. As I ran to get my equipment, I almost burst out crying in frustration and utter defeat in my belief that I had no reserves left for such an arduous task.

As our group ran through the camp gate, the one good thing was that it had finally stopped raining and the sun was trying to peek through the clouds. As we pounded down the road, a cloud of steam floated above the group from sweat and wet clothes. To our surprise, the attitude of the SAS corporals and sergeant totally changed from harassment to encouraging us to complete this last run. It was almost like they were different people.

The first few kilometres, thanks to their encouragement, my energy level seemed to increase. The pain around my blistered ankles and toes was just a dull ache, and I felt perhaps I was going to make it after all.

But another five kilometres further on and the pain of my blistered feet increased to unbearable proportions and at the halfway mark I decided I couldn't go on. Yes, I quit! I left the squad. The SAS corporal came back to me where I had sat down beside the road.

"You can make it, Sisson. You have come all this way, and it's nearly all over. Just 10 ks to go and you will have made it."

"I can't, Corporal. My feet are stuffed." He replied as he reached down and helped me to my feet.

"Here's something I was told that got me to the finish line on my selection course. Say to yourself that you will run just one more k. and then you will quit. When you reach it, you decide on just one more k. again. Then just repeat this after each kilometre and before you know it. You will be there. As I looked into his caring dark eyes, which I never thought I would ever see in such a tough veteran SAS soldier, I felt encouraged to keep trying. He continued. "Know this Sisson. When you are totally exhausted with not a single drop of energy left. You have used only 10% of all your reserves, which means you still have 90% left. A short rest and your body is fully revived. That is why SAS soldiers never run out of energy, ok?"

"Ok." I echoed back. Buck Paipa, this amazing Māori, gave me this most inspiring message that would carry me many times in the future when to keep going seemed impossible.

"Maybe I can do it!" I took three steps and my knees buckled from under me and I sprawled face down on the road, scrapping my knees and elbows. My body said 'no!' I sat up and looked down at my feet. My boots were full of sweat and – Oh hell, blood trickled out of my upended boot. Buck saw this.

"Take off your boot and let me look at your feet." He commanded. I undid the laces, slowly and painfully took off the boot and my socks were saturated with blood as I carefully rolled them off, revealing bleeding raw flesh around the ankle where blisters had once been.

"Shit." He said and ordered me to take the other boot off and also showed a similar condition around my toes.

"You stay here, and I'll get a Land Rover to take you to the camp hospital." I nodded. "You are off the course, but you have done well to make it this far. Try again next year." He ran off to catch up with the rest of the group. As I watched him run into the distance, my only thought was. 'That's it. Maybe I failed but I gave it my best shot.'

Later that afternoon, fourteen of us stood for the ending parade to prepare for the announcement of who had passed.

"Step forward when you hear your name called ..." Only seven names were called out and being read in alphabetical order, they called my name out last. I was so shocked that I didn't step forward for several seconds.

If I am honest, luck played a large part for me in passing this 10-day selection course. Some of those who finished but didn't pass, if luck had been slightly different, would have done so. Even some of those who dropped out if luck had been slightly kinder, they would also wear the SAS red beret.

I called it luck. Others might call it destiny, and others a self-generated reality, but who knows? In the coming years in Vietnam, this same luck/destiny, or whatever, was to show that in a split second of time, the slightest movement, the most fleeting thought, would make all the difference between living or dying. Life can so often be on a knife's edge and every decision, no matter how small, will have an effect that can last forever.

I am grateful that luck smiled on me that day. I will be forever grateful for this experience coupled with the inspiration of the SAS motto: *Who dares wins*.

3

THE SAS TRAINING AND UNEXPECTED PREPARATION FOR VIETNAM

Two weeks later, Major Mace (Commanding Officer) started his lecture by warning us we have probably let ourselves into something more than we bargained for.

"Over the coming year, we will train you for deep penetration behind the lines operations in Borneo." (So, the frequent 'behind enemy lines' comments were real after all). "As you know, Indonesia is in an undeclared war with Malaysia, who is an ally to New Zealand. We have New Zealand, British, Australian, and Gurkha Battalions protecting against any invasion from Indonesia. The job of the SAS is mainly reconnaissance, perhaps an ambush or possible 'hit squad' against key targets. You will be trained to be as highly effective as any 'Special force unit' possible."

The next 12 months were an intense training schedule in many fields. Morse code for signalling with secret codes, using the latest technology radio sets at that time. Kayak training more known as 'small boating' for operations around coastal areas, Cliff climbing, which scared the hell out of me, being not good with heights. The parachute training, in which I loved and eventually did 45 jumps, was a highlight for me. Weapon handling, which included many from the Soviet bloc and China. Demolition training, including explosive devices and booby traps, was part of the schedule. Unarmed combat was another favourite I enjoyed and joined a local Karate club to augment my skills. I got my 'Black belt' years later after I had left the army.

We spent the biggest amount of time in jungle training and living off the land. For that year, we spent every second week patrolling through rough New Zealand bush and became so at home in this natural environment and have loved camping and the outdoors ever since. Although it wasn't much fun during the winter months and was mostly wet and cold from the constant rain. The year of 1965 was the wettest I could ever remember.

'Shocker Shaw' was the main training instructor, and we all had a love/hate relationship with him. My most memorable instance was when I had two wisdom teeth removed by the army dentist as a precaution against toothache during operations. I was issued with a light duties card for the next three days, as any heavy exertion would cause my mouth to bleed. 'Wonderful,' I thought, meaning that I will get out of the 15-kilometre run in full battle gear that very afternoon.' I arrived back at the SAS orderly room, where most of the Squadron were lining up outside in readiness to start the forced march/run. I smugly walked up to 'Shocker Shaw,' handing him my light duty card, saying.

"The dentist has put me on light duties, because of having two wisdom teeth removed, Sergeant Major." He took the card, not looking at it, and instead looked hard at me. Then ripped the card into several pieces, dropping them back into my hand, saying,

"There are no light duties in SAS. If you were behind enemy lines with a bullet through your mouth, you would have to keep going. The enemies you will face don't take SAS prisoners. Get your gear and join the squad." I hated him and the dentist was right. After the third kilometre, my mouth bled heavily, and I hated him even more. Years later, I realized the important influence he would play in my time in Vietnam and will forever honour him.

Interrogation and torture training

Of all the interesting training courses, the one I gained the most from was the Interrogation and torture training. It gave me an understanding of the human mind in relation to fear that I could use in my future psychological work after leaving the army. However, within two years, I found myself in a delicate situation when this training came to my aid.

A psychologist from Auckland University had put together a five-day course in anti-interrogation and torture training, especially designed for the SAS. It was optional and only two of us signed up for it. As far as I know, they did not repeat this course for lack of interest, which was a pity because it was so valuable. Had it been my decision, it should have become standard training for all SAS soldiers.

It takes years to become proficient in interrogation techniques, so the first three days we only covered the very basics, while focussing on countering the effects of enemy intense questioning against us. What to watch for, what to say and not say. Keeping to your main story line and holding a certain attitude to give the impression that you know nothing of value that the enemy could try to extract from you, and much more.

The last two days, I found the most interesting, and we experienced being tortured with electrodes embedded under our fingernails, or toenails with sensors taped to parts of our bodies to monitor our responses. But we always had control and when it got too much, we could press a stop button. Thus, we could let the extent of pain stay within our own pain-threshold limits. This created a level of safety, giving us the confidence to experiment with levels of pain to gradually increase our pain threshold. Our tutor encouraged us to see how extreme we could withstand it. He also experimented with many different positions and levels of pain, ensuring that we never went beyond our extreme limit. But being in control removed any fear of being tortured and, as the day progressed, made it easier to withstand higher levels of pain, which totally amazed me. By the end of the fourth day, we were exhausted, and our tutor finished the day by asking:

"How would you feel if you had no control over the intensity of the pain and were totally at the mercy of your enemy to push you beyond all human limits? This question we will answer tomorrow."

The next and last day was the most enlightening of all, and our tutor started with a question:

"What do you think is the worst part of being tortured by a cruel and determined enemy?" Rogers answered, "The pain?" I nodded my agreement.

"No, not quite. The worst part is the fear of being totally at the mercy of your torturers, totally under their control. I remind you of the question of yesterday. When you feel totally helpless and a victim of their torture, this, in fact, makes the pain worse. In my research, between 60 to 80% of the suffering is from fear, from this sense of powerlessness. And this makes the pain more severe. When you are afraid you will be more tense, and this makes the pain worse. This is easy to understand if you think back to the last time you were emotionally upset. What was the worst part; the event that seemingly caused the feelings, OR the fear you felt about the event?" Seeing some confusion on our faces, he added.

"Okay, as you think of the event that last upset you, if you had no fear about it, would you have become upset?"

"I see where you are going with this. Of course, fear makes all situations worse." I commented.

"Exactly! You are getting it.

I want to show you a technique that puts you, the prisoner, back in control of the torture session, which means overcoming up to 75% of the suffering? Would that be useful to you?" We both nodded profusely. He continued.

"Not everyone can do this, and it is not for the squeamish, or faint-hearted, but as elite SAS soldiers, you both should be able to do it. In fact, anyone can do so if they have the determination to stay alive, withhold vital information from the enemy thus, saving many lives, or just determined to stay in control of oneself. So, are you ready for it?"

"Yes, sir," we both enthusiastically answered.

The technique to take back control from your torturers is to actually torture yourself and your own self-inflicted pain must be equal too, or more severe than the pain given to you by your tormenters. That way, you feel back in control of the entire process. Even though you are feeling twice as much pain, pain from them and pain from yourself, you are back in control, and this eliminates a huge amount of the total suffering, because as we have already discussed, most suffering is lodged in fear.

This technique is not about suppressing your fear or trying to get rid of it. To try would simply transfer the emotional pain into the subconscious and that would do huge psychological damage. It is about becoming the master of your fear. The key is by putting your complete attention on the exact spot where you are hurting yourself and so move your attention away from the pain of the enemy's torture."

Our tutor took a small bent nail out of his pocket and smiled.

"And here is the 'secret' weapon to take back control and reduce overall suffering by self-inflicted pain. As the enemy torture increases, you simply slip the bent nail into the palm of your hand, ensuring the enemy doesn't see it. See how I place it in my palm and simply by closing my fist and the tighter I clench it, the deeper the nail penetrates into the centre of my hand, where it really hurts. If the enemy torture is severe, which I imagine it would be, you need to break the skin and force the nail ever deeper into your flesh. The more it hurts, the less the enemy torture hurts. So, the more you hurt yourself, the more in control you are. The more in control you are, the less fear you have and so the pain from your tormentors diminishes in comparison. That way, you will never break because you are in control. You have become the master of the situation. Losing control is one of humans' greatest fears. The fear of losing control is a worse fear than even dying.

Seeing us both rub our faces nervously, he continued.

"I know on first hearing this sounds sick. But if your life is hanging in the balance, or the information you have puts the lives of many others at risk, it might be the only chance you have. I've never been to war, and I hope you never have to put this into practise for real, but if you do, it might save your life. British spies from World War Two and allied prisoners during the Korean War saved their lives and hundreds of their friends by withholding vital information from the enemy by this technique. Some carried their hidden nails on the inside of their belts, others in special canvas pouches up their rectum, but this carried the risk of infection of the wound in your hand. Others found nails in walls by extracting them and bending them about 90 to 100 degrees. Even the smallest nail works. Willing to try?"

Rogers wasn't so keen, but I had to do it just to prove I could. After putting some mild disinfectant on my hand, over the thirty minutes I learned things about myself, where I was mentally and emotionally weak and where I was stronger. At the beginning, while I had a stop button, I didn't have a powerful incentive to torture myself very much because I was still in control. Finally, with my consent, he removed my stop button with assurances that he would not go stronger than the extent of my already recorded pain threshold limit. He explained he would slowly increase the pain level and would signal me for the climax of maximum torture and to see how long I could endure it.

Then he started. As he slowly increased the pain, I knew I had to increase my own, and this resulted in an inner battle of resistance or to be fully present with my self-inflicted torture. The nail in my hand was really hurting, and I wanted to quit, but he kept giving me encouraging smiling glances to keep going. Finally, he gave me the signal of maximum torture. I could hold it for only 10 seconds before nodding, which signalled for him to stop. I felt disappointed in myself that I couldn't hold it longer, but he assured me I had done well and that this was still an artificial setting and, therefore, still had a built-in safety net. As he bandaged my bleeding hand, he continued.

"In an actual situation, the choice will be easier, as it will really be between life and death. If you choose life, not only will you overcome the pain, but also you will master your fear and the enemy will never break you. It is not about being strong-minded or with strong will-power. It is only about being fully focused with the energy in your hand, where the pain is. Nothing more."

Rogers asked:

"Is that why some mentally disturbed people physically mutilate themselves as a way to alleviate the mental pain?"

"Yes, that's right, it is the same principle. You find this with drug addicts and people with a lot of emotional pain. This is a vast subject I won't go into now, but to say that they use the physical pain to escape the mental pain. But this doesn't really work for them as they are using it to relieve or escape from pain, so no real healing happens. This technique we have been working with, it is not about escaping, but being fully focused on your self-inflicted pain to take back control of the situation and master your fear. Here lies the real difference. Even though it is the same principle, the focus and outcome are different."

This valuable experience gave me an understanding of how consciousness and the fear response worked. Not the torture itself, but in using my mind during reconnecting with painful memories and feelings I would face in the years to come.

What was helpful in this amazing psychologist, who, through the passage of time, his name has faded from memory, was not so much about taking back control or mastering my fear. Of course, these played a significant role, but the main reason it worked was because of our ability to be fully present with our own pain.

Years later, as I experimented with mental, emotional, and physical energies, our ability to be fully present with emotional pain, rather than focusing on the situations in life, was one of the major keys to releasing the fear and emotional trauma. Most people never go beyond their thoughts about the situation and how bad it was. Thus, they stay a victim to it and constantly seek a solution or to seek who is to blame. This only leads to more trauma and more pain. But when we find the courage to feel our feelings, healing happens.

But back in 1966, my youth eventually caught up with me and when the next detachment was formed for operations in Borneo, I was not chosen. I was simply too emotionally young to appreciate the dangers and seriousness of the tasks for highly trained and mature men in those dangerous, behind the line missions in Borneo. It was the right decision the SAS made not to send me and was more for my own safety and for those around me, something I was to understand when I got to Vietnam, 19 months later. In my disappointment after 15 Month›s training with the Squadron and having amassed a good deal of survival and self-management skills, I applied for a transfer to the Infantry Battalion already in Borneo and knew I would be guaranteed an overseas posting. I was more than keen to apply my skills, if not with Special Forces, then as an infantry soldier.

4
VIETNAM

From 1980, as I slowly healed from the horror of Vietnam to my return to that country in 1993, twenty-five years after my tour, the following story unfolded over many Breath Integration sessions. As I breathed and contacted suppressed memories, feelings of anger and fear, having been buried and totally blanked out by the subconscious for so long, were now resurfacing with complete recall. My tortured mind could reflect impartially on horrendous events, and then get swept up and lost in them again as fresh memories were released. As I breathed and paid attention to my feelings as to my practitioner's coaching, my mind became flooded with the lost memories from all that time ago: the hardships, the fear, the serious times, and the less serious.

* * *

Major Worsnop, our commanding officer at our base in Malaysia, looked carefully around the room at the 170 men of V2 Company assembled for their final briefing. At the conclusion, he finished with.

"You have trained well, and I have no doubt that you will give a good account of yourselves in the coming tour of duty." He suddenly paused, frowned, then sternly continued.

"By the way, I have this military police report from Singapore, where I know many of you spent your last leave recently. Who were the idiots who set off the thunder flashes'* down Boggy Street?"

---

* 'THUNDER FLASH: *A large firecracker that explodes loudly, but reasonably harmlessly, used in army exercises to simulate hand grenade and mortar explosions.*

We all looked guiltily at each other, knowing we had all had a part in the fun in Boggy Street. Then, with a smile, he continued.

"So, if no one is going to own up to it, when I establish your battle honours, it seems that I will have to include Boggy Street."

The room erupted in laughter.

ARRIVAL IN VIETNAM

As we walked down the ramp out of the back of a C130 transport aircraft, Danny McPhail, one of six platoon radio operators, began to furiously karate chop the surrounding air. "Let me at them. Let me at them," he yelled. We all laughed, and a group of Americans standing nearby were equally amused.

Our first view of Vung Tau air base was impressive. Hundreds of aircraft of every kind neatly parked, each individually surrounded with a wall of sandbags for protection from incoming enemy mortars and rocket attacks. The whole air base was a hive of activity, with aircraft and helicopters arriving and taking off every minute. Many American and Australian personnel were busily going about their business. The South Vietnamese flag of yellow with three horizontal lines fluttered in the distance at the camp entrance.

We were V2 Company, fit and enthusiastic and glad to be finally in Vietnam, after twelve months of jungle warfare training in Malaysia. We were professional soldiers, and all volunteers. I held a firm belief – one which would change years later – in the '*evils of Communism.*' Yet, it was real then, and I was here to do my duty in the fight against the 'antiChrist'. Russia, we had been told, was the instigator of the war in Vietnam. Russians were our real enemies. The Vietnamese were mere puppets in the global expansion of the Soviet Union, and back then, we believed it.

"V Company, fall in", our company sergeant Major Faulkner, bellowed, ordering Four, Five and Six Platoons to assemble in parade. All our equipment was checked. SLR rifle, seven magazines of twenty rounds each, eighty-round belt of extra ammunition for the section M60 machine gun, webbing, light pack, two high explosive hand grenades (US M26), one smoke grenade, claymore mine*, bayonet, machete, four filled water bottles (some carried up to six) first aid kit, emergency rations,

---

* CLAYMORE MINE: *These were flat, oval-shaped weapons with a high explosive charge compact with hundreds of ball-bearings that destroyed everything in the path of their blast. They were terribly effective in ambush positions against the VC.*

and an array of personal effects and spare clothing. In all, weighing approximately 36 Kilos (eighty pounds) of weight in combat gear. While others (radio operators, Machine gunners, and M79 grenade launchers) as much as 50 Kilos (110 pounds). Physical fitness demanded the highest level to be carrying this weight for up to 10 hours per day, moving slowly (approximately 500 metres per hour) through jungle terrain in hot tropical temperatures. Beside this, we possessed a kitbag of extra clothing and personal items to be held back in our base area.

It was November 1967, and no one knew what lay ahead. Each soldier stood silent with his thoughts, excitements, and fears. I looked around me at the assembled young men. A high percentage of them were Māoris** in the prime of their physical fitness. For the next six months (the length of our tour) these strong and young men were to live up to the warrior tradition of their ancestors, especially their fathers of the 28th Māori Battalion of the Second World War, demonstrating incredible courage. To be surrounded by these men was very comforting.

"Okay, each platoon, when dismissed, will get into those Chinook helicopters as designated by the flight crews." The Sergeant Major paused for a moment.

"This is it, chaps, we're here. Good luck. Attention! Diss – miss."

We clambered aboard the largest helicopter I'd ever seen. Each Chinook had M60 machine guns sticking out, it seemed, in every direction.

"How much weight can this thing carry?" I yelled over the sound of the chopper engines to the American machine gunner, who was standing next to me, peering out of his porthole.

"As much as you can fit into it, man," he smilingly yelled back, in a broad Texan accent.

An hour later, we landed at 'The Horseshoe,' so called because of its shape. Being the only hill in the area, it overlooked the surrounding countryside of mostly dried rice paddy fields. It was a heavily defensive positioned firebase that was commanded by a company of infantry protecting an artillery battery of 105 mm guns and a section of 81mm mortars. It was surrounded by barbed wire, and a minefield, set by the Australian engineers. Inside the basin-shaped centre were Company Headquarters and the guns.

On the high ground, looking outwards and surrounding the basin, were the bunkers, which were little better than holes in the ground, heavily

---

* Māori: *Native of New Zealand with a strong warrior tradition.*

sandbagged. Three men shared each bunker, ours having a 50mm heavy machine gun pointing towards the south-east. We could see the coast, about ten kilometres away to the east. The American Sixth Fleet was out there somewhere and became visible from the flashes of its big guns aboard the battleships and heavy cruisers, when they were called upon to provide supporting fire. To the west, a kilometre away, was a small Vietnamese village, 'Dat Do.' It was surrounded by a barbed wire fence, with two checkpoints at either end, and protected or guarded by a platoon of 'ARVN' (Army of South Vietnam) troops. These soldiers were poorly trained, undisciplined, and unmotivated. On two occasions in the middle of the night, they had running gun battles among themselves and with the locals, actions which caused us to go on full alert and 'stand to,' thinking that a Viet Cong attack was in progress. Dat Do was pro-communist: thus, the checkpoints and the concentration of troops around it. When we were not patrolling the surrounding countryside, the Horseshoe was to be our home for the next six weeks.

On our arrival at the Horseshoe, we were greeted by Lieutenant-Colonel Charlesworth, the commander of the Australian Battalion of which we were now part: The Second Royal Australian Regiment (2 RAR). With W Company, the other New Zealand infantry unit, a month later in December, the formation became known as the Anzac*[*] Battalion. We then comprised two New Zealand and four Australian infantry companies. With the other New Zealand units – 161 artillery battery, mortars, engineers, medical units and later the SAS (Special Air Service) – New Zealand was well represented.

The Colonel welcomed us and spoke mainly about the tradition of New Zealanders as elite soldiers who had fought beside Australia, their closest ally over the last seventy years, from the Boer War until the present day. We were very inspired and eager to get on with the job and prove ourselves in combat.

The next month, however, proved to be anything other than exciting, thanks to endless and fruitless patrols known as 'search and destroy missions.'

Manning the checkpoints around Dat Do village was very boring and hot. The monotony was broken only when a pretty Vietnamese girl

---

* ANZAC – *The Australian and New Zealand Army Corps, born out of the landings of the Australian and New Zealand forces at Gallipoli, Turkey in World War One in 1915, They have been honoured for some of the most courageous individual acts in the annals of modern warfare, while forging the ANZAC tradition.*

came through. The blokes would rush out from their shelter to be first to check her identification card (ID) and practice some limited Vietnamese language.

The attitude of the local populace was not good towards us. It was plain to see that they despised us, regarding us as an oppressive enemy. This surprised me, as I was certain we had come to Vietnam to defend the country against the invasion from the north, motivated by Moscow, so we had been told.

One afternoon while manning the checkpoint, a young Vietnamese child of about seven years, close to the age of my young brother, Grant, came up to talk to me. We couldn't understand each other verbally. I gave him some chocolate from my ration pack, and we had some fun communicating in sign language. Minutes later, an ARVN sergeant came and chased him away. I stood up, protesting.

He turned to me and, in broken English, explained.

"No Kiwi, you not understand. Often Viet Cong use young children to engage allied soldier in talking, while planting hand grenade beside them. Many Americans killed this way."

I nodded my understanding and felt sad that children were part of this war.

On another day, the monotony was broken when, while I was resting in a nearby tin shed, a bullet passed through the shed just above my head, causing a huge reaction of panic in the many bullocks passing through the checkpoint at that moment. An ARVN soldier in the next room had been cleaning his rifle, and accidentally fired off a round while reassembling his weapon. I ran outside, rifle in hand, to an enormous noise that had erupted. People and animals were running in all directions. Several bullock carts had stampeded through the barbed wire, close to some thatched houses and fences. Drivers were falling off. Loads of firewood and produce were falling off, and one cart had tipped over. Despite nearly being shot by the inexperienced ARVN soldier, I stood there amused at the total bedlam that was happening in all directions. I was, however, a little worried that people would be trampled on by the large panicking bullocks, and that the animals would injure themselves on the barbed wire fence.

Then, one of our guys, a sheep farmer from Canterbury in the South Island, knew exactly what to do. He calmly walked into the middle of the chaos of dust swirling around him, whistling loudly as if to his sheep dogs. The stampeding animals and panicking farmers magically responded to him as he majestically calmed their fears. As I watched him, I heard in my mind the soundtrack from the Clint Eastwood film 'The good, the bad and the ugly,' which highlighted in my mind his amazing calmness over this crazy situation. Within minutes, all was calm and peaceful again. We all shed tears of laughter, but also with great admiration for his calming ability on people and animals.

On one of our patrols, we had an ARVN officer accompany us to act as an interpreter in questioning locals or captured enemy. His English was excellent with a strong American accent, which he had gained whilst training in the United States. At one of the breaks, we talked for a while. I jokingly taught him to speak some words with a kiwi accent rather than American and some English 'Kiwi' slang words, much to the amusement of both of us.

On a more serious note, he told me how much the ARVN hated the Communists and would rather kill them than take prisoners. It seemed that half the South Vietnamese population were more bitter towards their own people in the north than they would have been against a foreign invader. I sensed a fear in his speech, and I detected this same hatred and fear in most of the ARVN I saw.

It was common for ARVN soldiers to run, even desert during battle. Because of this, the Americans brought in a policy that their wives and family live with them in their bunkers. They were then less likely to run and leave their wives to their fate to the enemy. I felt sickened at hearing this. Though I hadn't yet seen any action, this war was already sowing seeds of doubt in my mind, as well as challenging some of my values.

Every night in the Horseshoe, the intermittent firing of the 105mm guns interrupted our sleep. These would blast away for up to twenty minutes at a time, and sometimes for two or three periods throughout the night, giving fire support to some unit in the field that had just sprung an ambush or engaged in a firefight against an elusive enemy. Occasionally during the day, US air strikes were made against enemy positions, north-east of the Horseshoe about five kilometres away, in an area of jungle known as 'Long Green'. These attacks were made mostly by Phantom fighter bombers and were very impressive. Long Green was an area where several main line Viet Cong (VC) regiments were known to be based and most enemy attacks and infiltration in this district eventuated from here.

I spent a couple of days in Nui Dat, on an administrative task for Company Headquarters (HQ). Nui Dat was the main Australian Brigade camp, about seventy kilometres south-east of Saigon, and comprised three Australian infantry battalions with all supporting arms: approximately

5000 men in all. I was shown where our company tents were, as we would move to Nui Dat in a few weeks. Each tent could hold four men and had sandbagged sides for protection from VC mortar and rocket fire. What comfort compared with our bunkers at the Horseshoe that we could look forward to.

While there, I met up with some Kiwis from 161 artillery battery. One of them, Bobby Dennis, a Māori with a humour that kept me laughing for most of the time spent in his company. He gave me a tour of the entire camp, then with a couple of others drove me out of the camp beyond the wire barricades into no-man's-land, where they had buried an old ammunition box with bottles of whisky and rum. I was nervous about the obvious dangers, but they insisted we were safe. After several 'tots,' and back inside the protection of the camp, we spent the rest of the afternoon getting very merry. They took me back to my tent, totally drunk. This had been a wonderful break in the usual routine.

On my return to the Horseshoe two days later, VC activity around our position had become more frequent with each passing night. We stepped up our own patrols and ambush missions. It was as if they were checking us out thoroughly, perhaps for some future attack. We were constantly warned not to take chances and expose ourselves outside our bunkers. The danger of snipers was always present and going to the mess tent presented some concerns until a trench was dug by a work detail.

One morning, one of our patrols found a note tied to the wire near the entrance to the Horseshoe, written in poor English:

"Better stay awake Kiwi, because we come soon and you all dead."
We discussed several replies over breakfast. The best one I think was:

"Dear Charlie*. It would delight us to receive you. Please come at your earliest convenience. Dress formal. V Company."

One night a week later, the VC attacked the ARVN police station in Dat Do with rocket and machine guns. Eight ARVN were wounded, and one killed. A week later, the VC attacked the police station again, but this time they also attacked the Horseshoe directly opposite the station, where Five Platoon was positioned. Then withdrew, leaving Five Platoon and the very frightened police firing at each other. After several minutes, Five Platoon realized what was happening and stopped firing. The police quickly followed suit. It was a good VC trick, but fortunately, only one ARVN soldier was slightly wounded. A local water buffalo wasn't so lucky.

---

* Charlie: Nickname for the Viet Cong.

Each night every man spent two hours on sentry duty, commonly known as 'picquet' thus getting at best only six hours of sleep. I found this hard to adjust to.

Nightly VC activity continued to increase around the Horseshoe so much that an Australian battalion stepped up daily patrols in the area from Nui Dat to provide extra protection.

V Company also increased patrolling, and we started to find VC propaganda leaflets in English and colourful pictures describing the final Allied defeat in South Vietnam. It felt like something big was going to happen and some joked that Charlie had accepted our invitation after all and would be coming soon.

On several occasions, we came across VC camp sites that had been occupied only minutes before we arrived. Despite their increased presence, though, we could not locate and pin them down to a fight. This caused much frustration and tension amongst many of the guys.

One day when our platoon of thirty-six of us was returning to the Horseshoe from a patrol, a passing spotter plane (Bird dog) reported that a VC unit of company strength – three times our size, had crossed the road thirty minutes after we had passed by. They had probably been watching us and could have wiped us out if they had wanted to. Something is brewing, and little did we know that within two months the Communist Tet Offensive would erupt – the biggest campaign of the entire war.

In an early morning briefing, Sgt. (sergeant) Whitworth outlined the rules of engagement in a firefight with the enemy. He emphasized we must not discriminate when returning fire. "If it's a woman, or a child, fire back with everything you've got. Charlie is even using kids against us, the bastards."

Are we here defending the world against an oppressive invader who wants to take over the world, enslave us to their ideology and rape our women, the usual party line of the American propaganda machine, against the Soviet Union? Or are the Vietnamese so desperate that they will fight for their land using every resource available, including their women and children? I was not sure this was what I had signed up for. For the first time, I began to seriously question what sort of war I was involved in? As time passed, I was not going to like the answer!

5
LONG GREEN

We were now into December and the days rolled monotonously into each other. Dave Kingi, our acting Section Commander, put only one man at a time on sentry duty at night for one hour, rather than having the normal two men for two-hour periods. This was prompted to rest us, because of the increasing eruptions of bad tempers from lack of sleep.

One night, while on sentry duty, I was in a forward bunker close to the wire, when at 1.15 am, I suddenly heard excited muffled voices about thirty metres to my front. One was a woman speaking loudly in Vietnamese. I woke up Steve Vautier, and 'Grease Gun' (nickname for J. Tauhinu) who were sleeping in the same bunker. They alerted the rest of the section. The observation post behind us spotted three VC through the starlight scope, close to the wire. The starlight scope was a device like a binocular that enabled you to see the area almost as if in daylight. Shortly after, mortars fired some flares, illuminating the whole area. Charlie had gone. We opened up with machine gun fire and peppered the area with M79 grenades. The next morning, we patrolled the area, but there were no signs of the enemy.

On Friday, December 8th, just before darkness set in, Six Platoon moved out of the Horseshoe towards Long Green. We patrolled for three hours, arriving close to the centre of this very dense stretch of jungle, where we set up camp. Shortly before dawn the following day, we set off and continued to the far side of Long Green, and then patrolled back by a different route. On the way, we passed through a black water swamp that was waist deep. We couldn't see where we were stepping, and hell knows what was in it, or what we might step on. Such swamps throughout Asia often contained water snakes that were venomous. Leeches were more common and quickly attached themselves unbeknown to you, as you could not feel them biting and latching on to feast on your blood. The Bull leeches were more worrying, as they were many times larger and three of them could suck up to a pint of blood in an hour. After emerging from a swamp, each man carefully examined his whole body for such unpleasant creatures. I found three smaller ones that had somehow slithered into my pants and attached themselves to my legs. Not being able to pull them off as the wound would become infected, I lit a cigarette and safely burned them off before the platoon moved on.

"Hey Sas." (My nickname, that was derived from my previous service with the SAS). "Look at this." Bill Taare whispered and pointed to the side of the track where a huge yellow snake sat staring at us from the centre of its coils. I moved closer to get a better look, but Bill touched my arm. "Stay back. It looks dangerous and I think it's ready to strike." he whispered.

I'd seen plenty of snakes while training in Malaysia, but this was one I'd never seen before. It had the unmistakable diamond-shaped head, that showed it was venomous. I nodded, and we moved on. The whole platoon passed within two steps of it, each warning the man behind of the lurking danger, while it stayed unmoving, but threatening, with its unblinking stare.

That night nearly ended in disaster. Nearly every night, the platoon would set up an ambush position, manned by three or four guys with a machine gun and claymore mines. It was generally on a track close to a bend, where the maximum of enemy casualties would happen when it was sprung. At 3 am, having finished our stint of ambush duty and relieved by our replacements, three of us quietly moved back to the Platoon position, with me leading. Unfortunately, in the dark, I missed the track that led back. As quietly as possible, I pushed myself through the undergrowth in the direction where I was certain the Platoon was situated.

"You're going the wrong way Sas."

"No, I'm sure this is the direction to the platoon," I whispered back. I pushed through some undergrowth into a clearing, only to suddenly freeze on hearing the unmistakable click of a safety catch two metres in front of me. "Halt!" I heard the command in muffled English. "Don't fire, it's me, Sas," I frantically hissed into the blackness.

"Sh_t." Came a whispered voice that I recognized as Blue Neame, our section's machine gunner.

"You frightened the living sh_t out of me. Christ, you're lucky. I nearly opened fire."

I sat down beside him and Joe Hoani, his number two. We looked at each other in the dark without further speaking, realizing how close we had been to a tragedy. A high percentage of our casualties in V Company during the coming months were tragically from friendly fire. Arriving at my shell scrape and bed roll minutes later, I was thankful I was still alive, with a tinge of guilt that I also nearly cost the lives of my mates.

Blue Neame was a tall and well-built red headed South Islander. I had always liked Blue, even though he had once punched me in Malaysia while he was drunk, not recognizing who I was. We had been friends from when we first met fifteen months earlier before leaving New Zealand. He was always in trouble with the military police, generally for drunkenness and insubordination. Blue had little time for discipline, organisations, or tradition. Yet, what he lacked in traditional soldiering, he more than made up for in courage and combat skills. In the Months ahead, I was to be glad to have Blue around when the fighting started.

The next day, the three sections of the Platoon went off on separate patrols to cover a wider area, and in midmorning came across several VC tunnels and bunkers. We were ordered to destroy them. As the Platoon's booby trap specialist, training I'd receive back in Malaysia and prior to that with the SAS, I carefully checked them for the dangerous devices and for signs the VC placed to warn their comrades such as a piece of grass tied into a knot and other signals. Having been satisfied they were clear, I carefully climbed into one and began filling it in with my shovel. I wasn't strong enough to lift a large supporting beam that held the roof.

"Hey, Tua, give us a hand, will you?" I called.

Tua Hunter and Joe Hoani, two strong Māoris, climbed into the narrow hole and the three of us grabbed the beam and heaved upward, trying to dislodge it. Suddenly I saw the largest spider I had ever seen, about the size of my hand, fall from the beam and land at our feet and immediately jumped up onto my leg.

"Lookout," was all I could yell. The three of us desperately tried to scramble our way out of a hole big enough for one, climbing over each other, falling back in, and finally struggling out. Wide-eyed and alarmed, the other two looked at me for an explanation for my sudden warning, thinking it might have been a booby trap. I pointed, laughing, to the bottom of the hunker where the poor spider had been trampled. The rest of the section was sitting on the ground, holding their bellies, laughing at our comical 'Keystone cop' performance and our discomfiture.

We continued patrolling for the next six days, making eight days for the operation. During this time, we suffered from rationing and a severe water shortage. We could stretch out our food, but it was hard to have our water restricted in those hot conditions. It was the dry season in Vietnam, so we had little prospect of finding a stream with fresh water. Our base was reluctant to send any in by helicopter for fear that it would reveal our position to the Viet Cong. So, we were restricted to drinking only. Even cleaning our teeth, or washing hands and faces, was forbidden.

Two days in a row, several US C-130 aircraft flew low over us, spraying Agent Orange, the defoliant, to destroy the jungle and deprive the VC of cover from our spotter planes. The poison rained down on us in a thick mist and little did any of us realize how deadly it was. It eventually killed the vegetation and caused many deaths and future deformity in newborns for the local Vietnamese people for the next 20 years. It also was the major cause of cancer among our guys over the coming 50 years.

One day, a New Zealand journalist joined us for a day patrol, and afterwards commented on how safe he felt with us. For several days and nights, we set up ambush sites, but no VC walked through them. Then one day three VC were seen in the distance. We gave chase, but they lost us in the thick jungle. On another occasion, one of our blokes had a lucky escape, when without thinking, he picked up an unexploded butterfly bomb. These small bombs were dropped by American aircraft in their hundreds over a wide area, and they exploded on impact. Occasionally, one or two would fail to explode and could later detonate by the slightest movement.

"Put that bloody thing down," someone yelled. He threw it away and on landing, sat there for about 5 seconds and then exploded.

"Oh bloody hell," was all he uttered. It further showed that danger was at every turn, and we were to learn that casualties mostly happened when a person was mentally off daydreaming and not present. While on patrol, there was no time to let down your guard and relax.

On the sixth day, we were ordered to dig in and hold the position we were currently located. It had been discovered that a large enemy unit was in the area and, as there were only thirty-six of us, we had to take up a defensive position until Five Platoon could join us the next day. It was thought that they knew of our position and were moving towards us. The jungle was not so thick with visibility of about 30 metres.

Throughout the rest of day, a spotter plane 'bird dog' flew almost continuously overhead, trying to spot them. Finally, it did, and a heavy barrage of artillery fire erupted only five hundred metres away from us, and continued for over an hour, showing how close they were. We waited on full alert, expecting at any moment to see a large formation of VC, charging at us through the dust and smoke. There was no sign of them, and I wasn't sure if I was relieved or disappointed.

Intelligence later learned that the enemy unit was probably VC 25th Company moving towards its launching off position for the coming Tet Offensive and would have been avoiding all contact with Allied forces. So, we were in no real danger of being attacked, but none of us knew that.

Early the next morning, Company HQ informed us by wireless that 5 Platoon was close to our position, but ordered us not to wait for them, but to move towards the Horseshoe and home and 5 Platoon would follow suit. But moving undetected from the VC might prove difficult. The large VC unit reported the previous day had again disappeared. Even if it had been mauled by the artillery strike against them, it still offered a danger to a small unit as ourselves.

Half an hour later, having patrolled through open and exposed light bush, we came to a river. We replenished our much-needed water bottles, and then waded down the river, which offered better cover, for about a kilometre to where the jungle was much thicker. We dragged ourselves out soaked, muddy, and chilled by the coolness of the river and the morning air.

After a quick hot brew, we moved on through the thickest jungle encountered so far in Vietnam and, an hour later, reached Highway 23, which led to Saigon. Just then, 200 metres down the road, we saw a lone VC walk out into the middle of the road. He suddenly saw us and started running for all he was worth. Dropping our packs, our section gave chase, but he soon disappeared into the thick jungle at the side of the road. After retrieving our packs, we set off for home, arriving four hours later, feeling totally exhausted. It was great to experience a shower, shave, a change of clothes, and a good meal after so long on field ration packs.

The next week, leading up to Christmas, we spent doing sentry duty around the Horseshoe, or on the checkpoint at Dat Do. On the 21st, elements of W Company, the other New Zealand infantry unit, arrived at the Horseshoe, fresh from Malaysia. They were to relieve us once the rest of their company arrived, and we were to move to Nui Dat after the coming operation. Among the new arrivals was Roger Hyland, a good friend of mine from my SAS days, two years earlier, when we were doing our SAS training together. It was great to see him again and catch up on the news from home and Malaysia.

Two days later, a call came through on the field phone in our bunker from Roger Haworth, our company clerk. Roger was English, and we had spent many good times together back in Malaysia.

“Hey Sas, how would you like to extend your tour here in Vietnam for an extra six months? I am, and it would be great if you did as well. Company Headquarters is looking for volunteers to stay on. What do you say?”

“Let me think about it,” I replied. I was torn between the frustration and pent-up emotions of wanting to see some action and my growing distaste for the type of war I was in. That night I had a dream that I was a soldier in the German army during the Second World War and I could see myself in the German uniform. I was told years later that this is a common dream, of being dressed as the enemy for those who are betraying their moral values. This is one interpretation and no doubt there are others. But for me, even then the symbology was clear. Yet still, my frustration and thirst for action won out. But more so was a justification to apply the skills received from two-and-a-half years of intense combat training. I signed up the next day.

Christmas came and went almost unnoticed, except that standing orders stated that despite the Christmas ceasefire, we were to fire on any VC in our area. I didn’t like that. I attended Mass on Christmas Eve, but I felt uninspired and a little depressed. Picquet duty around the Horseshoe, and the checkpoint at Dat Do, continued as usual.

On the night of the 26th, we were each given two cans of beer. Then Private Gaunt, Lt. Wilson’s batman, got, through dubious means, a full carton of twenty-four cans, and five of us gathered in our bunker to celebrate. We got rather carried away with our laughing and letting off steam, which resulted in Lt. Hamish Wilson investigating and putting us all on charge for excessive noise in a war zone.

Two days later, we were marched individually before the Company second-in-command, Captain Dudman, and tried for our crimes. I felt very belligerent and argumentative. I argued with an edge of anger in my voice that considering we had been on active duty for six weeks without a break, living under stressful conditions and in unbearable surroundings, the charge was ‘ridiculous’. Becoming very heated, and at one stage Warrant Officer Faulkner cut in, warning me that my manners were unacceptable in front of a superior officer. We were all given seven days confined from any recreation facilities or alcohol and I got an extra ten dollars fine for insubordination. This didn’t matter, however, as the next day we were relieved by the rest of W Company, and V Company set off towards Long Green on its first major operation at full company strength.

6

NUI DAT

It was just at dusk as we moved through the barbed wire corridor leading out of the Horseshoe. Each man had five days' rations, including extra ammunition, and was feeling the extra weight.

I stopped and looked back for the last time at the uncomfortable home we had lived in for the last six weeks. I was struck by the beauty of the sunset, which appeared even more striking when seen through the smoke of a grass fire that had been burning much of the day around the Horseshoe. As we moved out, the fire had reached the minefield and the mines, along with the booby traps, were exploding every few minutes. As we patrolled through dried paddy fields towards Long Green, the sound of the mines gradually faded. Around midnight, we reached the edge of Long Green and camped just inside the jungle fringe.

The next day, December 29, 1967, Six Platoon left the company position to patrol a section of Long Green jungle in which Viet Cong units had been seen from the air the day before. We travelled for a while through the dreaded swamps, bog and quickly became filthy. I found only one leech after emerging, but several guys had several bull leeches attached to them.

There were many fresh tracks, particularly those made by the unmistakable 'Ho Chi Minh' sandals worn by most VC troops. These sandals were cut out from used vehicle tyre treads and were popular with the enemy because they offered silent movement through the thick jungle. In contrast, our Issued Australian combat boots made scraping noises when inexperienced allied troops moved through such terrain. We prided ourselves that we could move as silently as our opponents dressed in black.

That evening we stopped, tired and very muddy, about three

kilometres northeast of the rest of V company. And while we prepared our shell scrapes* and meals, two section set up an ambush for the night.

Early next morning, I was leaning against a tree with a mug of tea in my hand, when suddenly the calm morning was shattered by several shots. These were closely followed by machine gun bursts, then claymore mines exploding, and what seemed like just about everything else, from the direction of Two section's ambush position.

"They've got something," someone yelled.

Rifle in hand, I dived for my webbing, but had trouble getting it on, as my hands were shaking from the excitement. We fixed bayonets and spread out in an extended line. On a broad front, we quickly moved through the undergrowth towards the sound of gunfire. My heart was pounding so loud, I was sure that the man ten metres to my left could easily hear it. The firing stopped, and we slowed our pace, expecting at any moment to come across bodies. We reached the ambush site, but no one was to be seen, dead or alive. As we continued to move forward, firing suddenly erupted on our right flank where Three Section was sweeping some sixty metres away. A few stray shots thudded into the surrounding trees, and we hurriedly hit the ground for cover. The firing stopped, just as artillery shells from our gunners in Nui Dat came whistling overhead, to land 200 metres away down the track where the VC had disappeared. Andy Cowie, our platoon radio operator, had called in the guns, and within one minute of the first shot being fired, 105mm shells were coming in aimed to cut off the enemy's escape route. Our gunners' rapid response was very comforting, knowing that in a major contact such support would go a long way to winning the day, as we would one day discover.

Dave ordered us back towards the ambush position, where Joe Hoani from Two section was sitting on the ground recovering from the shock of the attack.

"You okay, Joe?" Dave asked.

Joe shook his head.

"Shit that was damn close. The bastards nearly got us that time."

What happened, Joe?" I asked, sitting on the ground next to him.

"Well, we decided to change the ambush site, because in the morning light, we could see that the killing ground was not open enough. We couldn't see that last night when we set it up. Hey, thanks." He put the cigarette in his mouth that Dave handed to him, already lit.

---

* Shell scrapes. *A shallow hole to sleep in, below ground level as a protection from enemy fire and shrapnel.*

"Well, Steve didn't put a sentry down the track as normal when moving things around. Anyway, I was rolling up the claymore cable, and I looked up to ask Steve where he wanted the bloody thing to go. And 'f_cken' hell, there's two bloody Charlies standing just 10 metres up the flipping track, and the first one's aiming his AK47 straight at me. I'd left my rifle on the other side of the track, so I dived for it just as this bastard opens up, and the second bastard's emptying his f_cken' weapon at me as well. Then by the time I could fire back, Mitch (Mitchell) had turned his M60 (machine gun) around and was blasting shit out of the track, and Charlie f_cked off. Then IB (Paterson) fired off the claymores, but we didn't know where they were pointing, or anything. But bloody hell, man, we had to get fire down on those 'Sh_ts' before they cleaned us out. It was too close a call."

Walking away, I reflected on how lucky we were not to have lost anyone so far. At a platoon debriefing an hour later, three section claimed to have killed the VC who nearly shot Joe, but no bodies were found, and their claim was never confirmed. Nor were any bodies found from the shelling when we swept the area where the Viet Cong had disappeared.

For the next five days, we put in a series of ambushes around the surrounding area, but there were no further signs of our elusive black pajamaed antagonists.

Shells whistled overhead at frequent intervals throughout the day, on their mission of destruction, to support an allied patrol in contact with the enemy. This was a stark reminder that VC patrols were active in this area and to be constantly alert.

I experienced a nagging toothache for several days that added to the discomfort of the heat, weight of pack (5 days rations) and the extra ammunition, as well as the emotional strain. The toothache eventually disappeared, allowing me to be more aware of my other discomforts. It was like being back on the SAS selection course.

We were quite close to the coast here and surrounded by swamp. The water was very brackish and salty, with a strong smell of sulphur from rotting vegetation. Even with our water-purifying tablets still made it difficult to drink, but that was all the liquid we had.

I enjoyed spending time with Andy Cowie. We would sit and talk in whispers, as experience was beginning to teach us that one could never tell when Charlie might turn up. Andy had been a close friend throughout our training in Malaysia, and we had often gone on leave together to Singapore. Yes, we had both been involved in the thunder flash incident on Boogy Street on our last leave.

“I think the boss is putting the ambushes in too close to the platoon position,” Andy said, starting a new conversation. “The problem is that the noise from the guys preparing food can be heard in the ambush site. What do you think?”

I nodded my reply, adding, “Yeah, and if the ambush party got pinned down by a large force, so could the rest of the platoon for being so close. Do you think the boss would be open to any suggestions?”

“I don’t know.” Andy replied. “He’s a good officer in many ways, like he knows his job, and I think he’s got guts (courage). He should listen to his men more.”

I liked Andy and was often amused when he got very excited when trying to explain something serious. He would stumble over his words in his hurry to get them out and succeeded in making everyone laugh. But he knew his job and was to prove his courage many times in the months ahead.

The early afternoon of the 3rd of January, we moved through the swamp yet again (no leeches this time) and joined up with the rest of V Company. Two hours later, we assembled in groups of 7 men spread over an open area of dried paddy, waiting for our ride back home. 10 minutes later, we were picked up by 24 ‘Huey’ choppers crewed by Americans and flown to Nui Dat in close tactical formation. ‘What a way to go to war and return to base again. My Uncles fighting in Libya and New Guinea in the last war would have been so envious,’ I remember thinking.

For the next six days, we settled into our new home in Nui Dat. Most of the time was spent reinforcing the sandbags around our tents for extra protection from possible VC rocket and mortar attacks. I joined two section and a few other blokes also changed sections to be with mates they felt closer to. It was good to be with guys you trusted, because it was anyone’s guess what was ahead of us.

Barbed wire and minefields surrounded the base of Nui Dat, much like the Horseshoe, but on a grander scale. There were many bunkers and strategically positioned observation towers that were manned around the clock. An area several hundred metres out from the wire had been cleared of jungle, so that an approaching enemy would be clearly seen. This jungle clearance followed an attempt by a large enemy force of NVA (North Vietnamese Army) and VC units in August 1966 to attack Nui Dat. They were courageously repulsed by D Company of 6 RAR (6th Royal Australian Regiment) in the battle known as

Long Tan, so named after a village close by.

Our tents were nestled in a grove of abandoned commercial rubber trees. The whole landscape was covered with thick red dust, which I was told would turn into red mud during the wet season. Something to look forward to, considering that I had signed on for an extra six months.

We all attended a briefing for a forthcoming operation code named 'Duntroon.' It sounded impressive. 274 VC Regiment, comprising three light battalions (up to 2000 men at full strength) a highly active and competent force operating in this area had finally been located. The plan was that two Australian battalions were to surround them. Then, United States infantry units, supported by tanks and APCs (armored personnel carriers), were to attack and sweep through, driving the enemy into 'stop groups' where V Company and several other Australian infantry companies were to be deployed. I noticed on the map that we were to be placed right in the middle of 274's escape route.

"It looks like we're going to see some real action at last," my neighbor whispered to me. I nodded.

"It looks like it. It was probably elements of 274 that we nearly met up with and called in the artillery strike against several weeks ago in Long Green," I answered.

All the platoons were to be deployed two hundred metres apart, so that as the VC stumbled into one platoon, then would retreat into another, taking casualties with each contact from well dug-in ambush sites. It was a good battle plan, but would it work as well as expected?

7
FIRST ACTION

Early in the afternoon of January 10, 1968, V Company left Nui Dat aboard Chinook helicopters. We arrived near the operational area, close to an ARVN camp, formed a 'harbour position', for all-round defense and waited for further orders. Many Australian infantry troops moved past our position on their way to their designated 'jump off' positions for the coming battle.

"Gidday, Kiwi." Good luck to you guys," they would call out as they trudged past.

"How you're goin', Digger?" Stay safe!" we would reply.

'Digger' was an Australian soldier's nickname born from the gold mines in Australia dating back 100 years. We never mixed a great deal with the Australians while in Nui Dat, as the companies were isolated from each other. Also, there was some rivalry between our two forces, particularly back in Malaysia, where there were many drunken fights in the bars just outside Terendak camp, which housed the Australian and New Zealand Battalions. But, right then, in the common danger we all faced, there was a close brotherly connection we all felt towards each other.

At 7.20 the next morning, we clambered aboard the US Iroquois UH-1Ds helicopters (slang named 'Huey') the modern-day war horse. We were to be the first wave of troops to land in the operational area, under the support of massive artillery fire. Our job on landing was to secure the landing zone (LZ) for the rest of the incoming companies. We had been warned that VC units could be in the area, so each wave of helicopters could only be on the ground for only 5 seconds, max, just enough time for the troops to jump clear of them.

As we sat on the floor of our Huey, me in the doorway (so will be first out on landing) with its engines roaring, and rotor blades spinning, waiting for the final orders to take off, I looked around me. No doors on the helicopters, no safety belts, and throughout the war where thousands of Allied troops were transported this way, no one ever fell out, except when a Huey was shot down by enemy ground fire, which unfortunately happened from time to time. There were webbing straps protruding from the floor that we would hold on to with one hand when the chopper was in a step bend. It never occurred to us that there was any danger in this. We were more concerned about the danger that waited for us on the ground.

We were all laden down with our packs full of rations, extra ammunition, grenades hanging from our webbing, rifles in our laps, cocked with the safety catch on, ready for action. Strapped to our packs were M72 rocket launchers to be used against enemy bunkers. We were certainly well armed. I looked at the faces of my friends accompanying me. Some looked blankly at the floor, whilst others had their eyes closed, as each wrestled with his inner thoughts and feelings about the coming engagement. I thought about the danger I was in and was astonished that I had volunteered to come to this country where the killing of fellow human beings was the expected norm. My stomach was tense with a mixture of fear and excitement. Right then, I would have given anything to be back in New Zealand.

At last, the order was given, and the fifteen helicopters in our wave lifted off the ground together, banked sharply to the right and then straightened up in perfect battle formation. Forty seconds later, I looked back from the doorway and could see the second wave lifting into the air behind us. A further forty seconds after that, the third wave, and then the fourth, the fifth, and so on until the air was full of helicopters, each wave in close battle formation. I glanced at the ground sweeping past 500 metres below, and saw it suddenly erupt with massive artillery fire, with what seemed like hundreds of guns pounding the Viet Cong positions. My fear dissolved, and suddenly I felt highly ecstatic. It was as if I were in a cavalry charge, sword drawn, charging into the face of the enemy. I had felt a similar, but much less rush of adrenalin years before while playing rugby, charging into the opposition forward pack to form a ruck. But this was an excitement greater than I had ever experienced. I gripped my rifle tighter, eager to reach the battlefield and engage the enemy. I was determined to give of my best for God, Queen, and country: if necessary, I was ready to die if my time came.

At such moments, foolish men lose themselves to Mars, the mythical god of war, without the wise understanding of the consequences of their motives and actions. What lay ahead would be a valuable wake-up call for me.

Fifteen minutes later, our wave of Hueys descended into an open area of grassland surrounded by scattered jungle. This is it! The die is cast, and my fate awaits me. We landed with a bump, and I bailed out, closely followed by my mates. On clearing the chopper, I ran to the nearest cover, a termite mound, and dived behind it, rifle at the ready. When the wave of choppers took off, we quickly spread out, bent over, sprinting to all sides west of the LZ, watchful of any snipers. Having reached the edge of the LZ (landing zone), I threw myself behind a clump of bamboo, as the second wave came thundering in to disgorge another company. They then secured the other side of the LZ as the third wave came in. By now, we could be certain that there were no VC in the immediate area.

Over the next hour, waves of choppers continued arriving, unloading troops and back-up supplies for the coming battle. When the whole battalion had arrived, our position was relieved by an Australian company, and we set off towards our battle position. I was more than impressed by the organizing of such a massive operation by high command and logistic support. It was comforting to know that they knew what they were doing.

We travelled slowly our usual 500 metres per hour, not to give our presence away, through scattered jungle towards our objective, two days' march away. We all had total faith in our lead scouts, who had already proved themselves in the previous two months of patrolling.

Throughout the day there was a lot of shelling of 274's position. "The poor bastards", I remember thinking. Joe Runga, our section commander, swapped his M79 grenade launcher and sixteen launcher grenades for the much lighter M72 rocket launcher I was carrying. The extra weight caused me to feel tired by the end of the day.

That night VC mortars landed within 300 metres of us, and we heard the next morning that an American unit had suffered thirty casualties during the night from the VC mortar counterattack. No one in our company HQ knew how many were killed. We were under no illusions that this operation was going to be a pushover.

The next two days until we arrived at our ambush position, there were many fresh signs of VC movement through this area. We moved ever more alert, with the extra pressure on our lead scouts, as the threat from walking into one of their ambushes had been heightened.

The second day, while patrolling, I could see far in the distance an armada of Huey's, no doubt filled with Australian Companies moving towards their objective in the scheme of the coming battle. Suddenly one Huey dropped out of formation and plunged towards the ground. I whispered to the man closest to me.

"Shit, look!"

The Huey wasn't spinning (rear rotor blade not working) or tumbling, but just in free fall with its nose slightly lowered. Whether it had been shot down or through mechanical failure, being too far away to tell. It disappeared behind a distant hill and didn't see it crash. I lowered my head in reverence to the 4 aircrew and 7 soldiers, who probably all died a quick but terrifying death.

Late in the afternoon we finally arrived at our destination and the Platoon dug in, forming an all-round defensive position. Our section of ten guys were sent on a patrol to ensure there were no enemy close by and returning late, I didn't get the chance to dig my 'shell scrape'. I was so tired, having had only five hours of sleep the night before. After a quick meal, I rolled up on the ground and immediately fell asleep.

"Wake up quick. Charlie's in the area. Stand to." Sergeant John Whitworth, silently moving around and waking up each man. I rolled over, shook my head to wake myself up, and looked at my watch: It was 8.30 pm. With rifle at the ready, and grenade launcher by my side, I lay there staring out into the inky blackness, waiting for my eyesight to adjust to the night.

Suddenly, from Four Platoon's position about 200 metres away, heavy firing shattered the stillness of the night. I regretted not digging a shell scrape and felt very exposed. Shadows danced across the jungle in front of me, but they were only my imagination. Gripping both weapons tightly, I slipped off the safety catch on both. If Charlie came bursting through the bush in front of me, I'd have about one second to get them before being overrun. I slipped my sweaty left hand from holding the stock of my rifle, and slowly gripped my right hand that held the pistol grip, to stop it from shaking. I was barely breathing. Slowly, I took a deep breath, controlling the exhale in a long sigh, so that it made no noise. The closest man was ten metres to my right but could see no one and felt I was the only one on this whole battlefield to face the enemy on my own. I felt an inner conflict between excitement and fear.

Meanwhile, the firing from Four Platoon intensified, with many explosions from grenades, rocket launchers and claymore mines. To my relief, Sgt Whitworth crawled to each of us, giving encouragement, and to let us know what was happening. Apparently, a large VC unit had walked right into Four Platoon's position and was paying for it.

The firing began to subside, with only occasional shots ringing out. Then, from Five Platoon's position on the other side of us, and much closer, heavy fighting broke out. Flares from our artillery batteries were descending, creating an eerie light and shadows that danced on the leaves. The shadows I had previously imagined suddenly created a life of their own and seemed even more real. Sweat kept dripping into my eyes, causing me to blink continuously and affecting my concentration. From the light of the flares, I could see that my position offered very little cover. I crawled to my left and settled down behind a log, placing my rifle and grenade launcher in a convenient V-shaped cut on top of my cover. No sooner had I moved there than tracer* bullets thudded into the surrounding trees, some of them as low as half a metre above my head, stripping branches and leaves that showered down on top of me. The bullets made a distinct cracking sound as they passed close overhead and were very unnerving. The conflict inside of me to control my fear was far worse. A couple of blokes to my right opened fire, more from fright than from seeing anything.

I resisted the temptation to tie the thin black scarf from around my neck to around my forehead to soak up the sweat it was designed for, being too afraid to take my attention away from my immediate front. Then a shadow with real substance ran through the bush in front of us, only twenty metres away. Our machine gun team, Blue Neame and Toi Rawiri, opened fire with a long burst, followed by two short bursts, but missed.

The horrific sounds of battle from Five and from Four Platoon intensified as men on both sides were fighting for their lives. Lying here waiting seemed harder and more frightening than being involved in the firefight, something that got confirmed for me in the coming months. Waiting was the real mind destroyer. The noise was heightened by artillery shells that started crashing in around four and five platoons, trying to catch the enemy in the open. This added deafening sound somehow helped my personal inner battle.

It reminded me of an SAS lecture 18 months earlier. 'If you are thinking about whether you will survive the mission or not, prevents you from being present in the job in hand. Give up your hope to survive and just focus on the task. It controls the fear, and makes the job easier.'

In the chaos surrounding me, this thought helped me give up any hope

---

* Tracer Bullet*: Is a bullet that glows during its flight and can be distinctly seen. Its purpose is to show where an enemy target is located, so other rifleman can also direct their fire to that location. About every 5th round in a magazine was a tracer.*

of surviving this madness. The enormous amount of adrenaline pouring into my body transferred my fear into excitement, and manifested as a stirring of anger, bursting to express itself.

"Come on, you bastards, I'm waiting for you," I silently muttered. I was primed and ready. To my disappointment, the shelling suddenly stopped, then the firing from both platoons died down with only sporadic shots and they also eventually stopped. I glanced at my watch, and it told me it was after midnight and yet it seemed like only a few minutes had passed since being woken.

After that came a suffocating, oppressive silence that was more terrifying than the actual battle. Minutes dragged by and nothing stirred. My excitement was now losing ground to fear.

Suddenly, the uncanny silence was pierced by the horrible blood-curdling scream of someone obviously mortally wounded, about 50 metres in front of me. It sounded more animal than human and was followed by a more muffled scream accompanied by coughing that faded away to a deathly silence. I wanted to scream to myself as fear was winning over my excitement and held my breath to suppress all feelings. I dared not move, not even to shift position for comfort. "Keep looking to the front," I told myself. "Just keep looking to the front. They could appear at any moment."

I heard a rustle of leaves behind me and spun round to see Graham Peddie crawling up to me.

"You okay, Sas?" he whispered.

"Yeah. How about you?"

"I'm okay. Hey, that was bloody hot." I nodded in agreement.

"Did any enemy rounds come close to you, particularly close over your head?" I whispered back. Seeing him nod, I asked,

"Did they make a strange cracking sound to you?"

"Yeah. That was bloody unnerving. Probably breaking the sound barrier or something. I don't know."

We sat together, alone with our feelings, but each glad to have a friend close by. The silence was intense, and even the usual jungle sounds of insects had been stilled. I was to learn that I would never get used to this incredible quietness that always seemed to happen just before and immediately after a firefight. The tension was like a tightly coiled spring waiting to be released. Then, nature found the ideal tension reliever. Graham leaned towards me and whispered.

"Did you see anything before?"

"Yeah, but I didn't get a chance to fire. Did you?" I whispered back.

"Nope, didn't see a thing, but I sure opened up on the bastards." This remark had to be the funniest thing I had ever heard, and a giggle escaped out of my nostrils. That was enough to set us both off, and we rolled onto our sides, giggling into our hands to suppress the noise and the laughter. Paddy, our section 2 IC (second-in-command) crawled along to us.

"Hey, you bastards, shut up. There's nothing to laugh at. Five Platoon has had three casualties."

Graham and I looked at each other in the dark, and we both collapsed onto the ground, burying our faces in the red dust in hysterical, silent laughter. It was the perfect release. Later, after Graham had crawled back to his position, I felt refreshed and relieved, with my spirits restored. The rest of the night, half the platoon slept for two hours, while the rest of us 'stood to' on alert, and after two hours, we swapped over.

Early the next morning, Joe called us for a briefing.

"It sure was pretty hot last night. Four Platoon killed eight VC and Five Platoon got one. But their sweep of the area this morning revealed many blooded drag marks, so both platoons probably killed many more times that number. Unfortunately, five platoon suffered three wounded. Apparently, one was shot through the face and is seriously wounded. I don't know who the casualties are, but we'll find out later today. They're calling in a 'dust off'* this morning. Anyway, our job is to do a sweep around our position to look for any dead or wounded Charlie. The jungle's quite thick and so warning you that if we meet any of them, it will be at damn close quarters. So, fix your bayonets. Let's go."

We moved out in single file, then spread out in arrow formation. I had my rifle butt into the shoulder in the aiming position so that I could quickly fire. The M79 was under my left arm held there by its sling, loaded with a grenade ready to fire. If I had to, I could fire both weapons almost simultaneously. I felt calm, but my stomach was stirring as if something were about to happen.

Suddenly, Bill Taare, our lead scout, saw two VC, fired several shots, and ran forward. Joe followed behind him, shouting something. I was next and yelled, "Contact front," while sprinting forward. I was more able to use my rifle and bayonet in close contact fighting if needed. There was no fear; just a rage after weeks of tension, demanding to be expressed.

Suddenly, I glimpsed two black-shirted VC, 20 metres away through the jungle, but both Bill and Joe were in my line of fire. I sprinted through

* Dust Off: *A helicopter for evacuating wounded.*

the undergrowth to my right so I could get a clear shot, but had lost sight of them. Knowing the direction they had gone, I dropped to one knee, placing my rifle beside me, swung the M79 grenade launcher into my shoulder and opened fire. I fired six grenades ten metres high into the trees, so that when they exploded, they would shower the VC with wooden as well as metal shrapnel. The rest of the section had caught up and was also firing in the same general direction. They moved on through the undergrowth.

I was suddenly alone. Slowly standing up, crouched over, totally alert, and aiming my M79 at anything that might move. Still holding my gaze in front of me, I reached down, felt for and then carefully picked up my rifle and changed weapons for close quarter combat readiness. My rifle and bayonet might be more useful right now. Then my eyes fell on a VC only three metres away, lying down with his head against a tree, facing me. We saw each other at the same time. I aimed my rifle for the middle of his head. He was unarmed, didn't move, and we held eye contact. I then noticed that he was mortally wounded, with a large bullet hole in his face with part of his cheekbone jutting out of the hole. He made a feeble effort to sit up, but collapsed again. Blood was everywhere. Though revolted by the sight, I couldn't tear my eyes away. I could taste the bile in my throat and felt nauseous. He was obviously dying as he continued looking at me. He was making horrible moaning and gurgling sounds as spittle and blood formed hubbies around his mouth. His eyes glassed over as his head rolled onto his chest. This revealed the exit of the bullet from his face, causing a large part of the back of his head to be blown away.

"I must kill him, and put him out of his misery," was my only thought. Making a supreme effort, I moved forward, raised my rifle, and aimed my bayonet at the centre of his chest. As I did so, I heard Joe's voice beside me, who had reappeared with the section.

"Don't worry about him. Guard that flank, quick," he yelled. I snapped into action and ran over to a large rock he had pointed to. As I ran past the dying VC, Bill, who had shot him, was leaning against the tree, spewing up his breakfast. Five minutes later, a shot rang out as someone put a bullet through a fallen enemy. I was glad it was not me that finally had to do it. At that moment, I realised just how easy it was to die.

As I numbly walked back to our platoon position, I didn't know how to feel. Elated at surviving my first action, or disgusted at what I had just seen? I chose to feel nothing, and my feelings started to freeze. Yet, I couldn't stop sensing that something incredibly valuable had died in me, along with that VC. Perhaps some would call it innocence, but whatever the name, it was lost. Even though I hadn't physically killed the man, the split second I aimed my rifle and bayonet with intention, my body reacted as if I had. I could feel myself closing down to survive emotionally.

That day in Vietnam, a valuable part of me died.

8
THE 'MISSING' HELICOPTER

Later that morning, Lt. Hamish Wilson gathered us together for a platoon debriefing.

"Well done, men. The operation has been a success, according to this message from Battalion HQ. A good portion of 274 Regiment has been knocked out."

This was the news we had all hoped for. Wilson continued.

"All their RPG rocket launchers have been captured, as well as a mountain of weapons, drugs, ammo, food and a large quantity of Cambodian money worth about 1000 American dollars. More importantly, though, vital documents relating to 274's activities for the next twelve months have been captured. As a fighting unit, it is finished and out of the war."

The 274 Regiment did quickly rebound and took part in the coming Tet Offensive because of their effective logistics, supplied by the Ho Chi Minh trail. This was a military supply route of weapons, manpower, ammunition, and other supplies running from North Vietnam through Laos and Cambodia to their combat units in the South. The Americans on many operations tried to close this route, but each time, within a week, the trail was back open.

The platoon completed a wide sweep around our position. A lot of blood and blood-smeared drag marks were found, for it was the Practice of the VC to remove their dead from a battlefield to conceal their losses. They sometimes went into battle tied to each other, so that a fallen comrade could be easily dragged away, hidden, and later buried.

Four Platoon found another body that brought the number of confirmed kills for V Company to ten, not counting the estimated high number of dead and wounded that had been dragged from the engagement.

The sounds of fighting, particularly heavy shell fire from the direction of the battered 274's location, continued throughout the day, as we moved towards a resupply location. 'They're really taking a hammering,' I thought.

We were resupplied by helicopters with ammunition and American rations that were twice the size of the Australian ration packs. So, we were well laden, with bulging packs. The best arrival, though, was the mail from home. There was a letter from both my parents. Being in contact again with my family was such a joy. It was the first happy moment I'd had for some time.

The following day, we rested. It was great to read, write letters, play cards, and catch up on much needed sleep between sentry duties.

The next day had also been planned to be a rest day, but that was about to drastically change. Just after breakfast, as I lay beside my shell scrape, basking in the early morning sun before it got too hot, without warning, a claymore went off fifty metres away. Several shots followed the explosion. I rolled into my shell scrape, clutching my rifle. There was a brief pause, and then it sounded as if every weapon in Vietnam had opened up. I peered over the top of my trench with both my M79 and rifle at the ready. I couldn't see anything, as the battle was taking place behind some dense jungle, with the odd shot thudding into the trees behind me, prompting me to keep low.

"Sas. Sas. Come here, we need you." It was Joe yelling for me. I climbed out of my shell scrape, keeping low, with my M79 tucked in my shoulder, extra grenades in hand, and rifle slung under my left shoulder, I ran to where his voice came from.

"To Andy's trench, Sas. He can see the bastards." I sprinted over to Andy, on the far side of the platoon's perimeter, where he was firing sporadic shots as the Viet Cong withdrew.

"I missed them! Bloody hell, and they were right in front of me," he yelled in excitement.

"Where are they Andy?" I shouted back.

"Over there." He pointed to his left. I looked around for some cover. There was none; Andy's shell scrape was too small for both of us.

"Fire! They'll get away, quick, fire." Andy yelled, his voice hoarse with excitement.

"I'm a sitting duck here," I shouted back, panic rising. I felt the eyes of half the platoon boring into my back. I fired a grenade into the trees, where I glimpsed a fleeting black shirt. On reloading, my shaking hands caused me to fumble. My thoughts screamed at me that, if any VC within 100 metres looks in my direction, I'll be taken out as it's so open here. I fired two more grenades, then glanced at Andy.

"I'm finding some cover. See ya."

There was none in the immediate area. I sprinted back to my shell scrape and hurled myself into it, and only then I felt safe.

It was a good move as within minutes, enemy fire erupted again in another section of the Platoon perimeter, with rounds thudding into the surrounding trees. The Viet Cong had come back to have another go at us. I was thankful that I had followed my instincts and found cover.

"Sisson, here quickly, over here." It was Lt. Wilson. The curse of being the Platoon's grenade launcher operative. I peered over the rim of my shell scrape. Enemy bullets started kicking up the ground between me and Hamish Wilson's position. I ducked for cover. My heart was pounding as I struggled to stay in control.

"Sisson! Sisson!" His voice reached me through the sounds of the firefight. I carefully peered above the protection of my shell scrape and saw my platoon commander, his back to me, firing at the enemy with one hand, and waving frantically with the other, signalling that I run to him. Being closer to the enemy, his position offered a better field of fire. I looked at the twenty-metre clearing that separated us: an area that had been torn up by enemy bullets only seconds earlier. I felt nauseated, my throat constricted, and I could barely breathe. A thousand thoughts scrambled my brain, and I saw the mutilated body of the VC whom we had killed two days earlier. I imagined myself looking that way, which was to haunt my dreams for the next 5 years. On the verge of throwing up, I looked again at Hamish, who was now waving even more frantically. Resigning myself to 'whatever' outcome, while summoning every ounce of willpower, I forced myself to my feet and sprinted across the clearing. Throwing myself on the ground next to him, I unknowingly knocked my grenade launcher sights out of alignment. Taking quick aim, I fired off a grenade at a group of the enemy 30 metres away. With my sights out of plumb, the grenade hit a branch two metres in front and above me, bounced, hit another branch, ricocheted again, and landed just ahead of our guys to the right of us. It fortunately did not explode, as M79 grenades must travel a certain distance before they were armed.

"Hey, watch what you are doing", came a protest yell from several guys near where it landed.

I was terror-stricken and emotionally shattered. This was the last straw as my last remaining confidence drained away. Burying my face in the soft red dust, I silently sobbed, feeling my sanity abandoning me. Along with my departing sanity, all hope of physically surviving also left. My senses then seemed to pass through the terror and that nothing mattered any more. No hope, no nothing; just me and this experience. I noticed the sensation of terror in different parts of my body and felt these places out of interest, as I had never been so present with my fear. Noticing also that I was breathing deeper than usual and breathing in the red dust caused me to cough and choke. I lifted my head, wiped the dust from around my nose, mouth and further noticed that the breath was increasing a new type of awareness I had never had before. While fully embracing the emotions of fear, a new feeling of detachment from the terrifying situation unfolded and viewed myself as if I were looking at someone else, playing out a nightmare. To my surprise, the intense fear dissolved. Next came a feeling of inordinate calmness. Slowly, I refocused my vision and looked around. Everything was slowing down, moving as if in slow motion. Wilson was busy firing at the now retreating VC, as was the rest of the platoon, yet his movements when changing his magazine were like those in a slow-motion movie. No words could describe what I felt. The closest would be euphoric bliss. No horror, no anger, and no fear!

Deliberately readjusting my sights, I calmly began delivering grenades in the general direction of the jungle where the enemy had disappeared. As I reloaded and fired, I wondered at this strange phenomenon, and this thought seemed to speed things up to their normal speed again. As quickly as it came, this amazing sense of presence, or whatever it was, passed.

Heavy shellfire suddenly came screaming in, called in by Andy, who was Lt. Wilson's radio operator. Our gunner's calculations were slightly amiss, and the shells exploded only fifty metres away (far too close for 105 mm artillery). Wilson and I had no real cover, so we both covered our heads with our arms and hugged the ground. One shell landed less than thirty metres away and the shrapnel whizzed all around us. I peeped out from under my armpit to see Andy through the dust and smoke, frantically yelling into his radio, imploring for the shelling to stop before we were all killed. 'Well, if I'm to die here, let's hope it's quick,' was my only thought, with no sense of fear. Finally, the shelling stopped.

"A steel helmet would have been helpful, wouldn't you say, Sisson?"

"My bloody oath, sir," I replied.

"Well done," Wilson continued. "I think between us all we might have got them." He had not been aware of my intense drama, being so involved with the heat of the battle.

I felt a sense of satisfaction that I had, in some way, dragged myself from the depths of insanity, back to myself to effectively do my job. Then, I had a subtle and strange thought – 'I hope my grenades didn't hurt anyone!' Perhaps it showed a oneness with all life, that I was to explore in the years ahead, or a symptom of madness?

Three Section," Wilson called out over his shoulder, "Do a sweep to our immediate front," Looking back at me, he said, "Go and rest up. We handled that well."

"Thanks sir."

Three Section found one dead VC, and several blood-smeared drag marks. I settled back into my shell scrape, holding my face in my hands, wondering what had caused everything to slow down. I shook my head, to empty it of confusion. I dared not speak of it to anyone, concluding that it was a sign that I was going insane and didn't want to lose their trust in me to do my job. Or worse, be cassavaked out (extracted by helicopter) as mentally unfit.

Later, when I felt better, I wandered over to Andy to find comfort with a friend.

I've made an interesting discovery, Sas," he began. "It seems that in a close quarter firefight there's a tendency to fire high. It's similar to night firing. That's why I missed those Charlies'. I mean, they were right in front of me. A blind man couldn't have missed them!"

"Well Andy, I think we've going to get a few opportunities to put your theory to the test," I whispered back. It was a theory that was to be proved right.

The rest of the day, the guys rested. Some played cards, slept, quietly talked while others played practical jokes on each other. Some jokes were a macabre way of relieving tension.

Lou Phillips, the company medic, was acting strangely, rolling a sweet/candy tin around on the ground with his foot. His odd behaviour caught the attention of me, and BB (Bill Taare).

"What ya doing, Lou?" BB asked. Lou slowly picked up the tin and handed it to him, saying "Open it and help yourself to a lolly."

Bill opened it and exclaimed as he dropped it. "Bloody hell, Lou!" as a monstrous tarantula spider jumped out. I later had a practical joke played on me when I found a dead snake under my pack, placed there by Blue Neame after he'd killed it. To say I got a shock would be to put it mildly.

The next day, the 17th of January 1967, was quiet, and we continued catching up on some much-needed sleep that allowed our nerves to settle down. Mercifully, the practical jokes stopped at the urging of Lt. Wilson. The following morning, after filling in our shell scrapes, we moved out to join up with Five Platoon five hundred metres away.

It was the practice of VC patrols to move into an area recently occupied by Allied troops and search for anything left behind. Some American units, after being in one spot for a few days, often undisciplined, discarded unwanted equipment and food before moving on. Consequently, it was attractive for the VC to check out our campsites. Our plan was for 2 hours after moving out was to call for artillery to shell our abandoned position. This we did, and in came the shells from the big 155mm American guns in Nui Dat. But the gunner's calculations from our instructions were in error and they brought the first few shells close to our current location instead of our abandoned position. This was the second time in two days we were under fire from our own artillery. With shrapnel whistling all around us, we hugged the ground. I placed my pack over my head for extra protection. Most trees around us were stripped of their leaves. Within a minute, the shelling mercifully stopped. It was a miracle that no one was hurt. I wondered how many casualties had been inflicted from such so-called friendly fire by allied troops during this war, or for any other war.

For the next three days, V Company patrolled back towards our arrival LZ (landing zone), where we were to be picked up by helicopters and flown back to Nui Dat. We travelled by a different route, winding our way through some very dense jungle. It was hard going, particularly for the lead scouts, and each night, we collapsed exhausted. This made it particularly hard to stay awake at night during sentry duty. We would sit or lie manning a machine gun in pairs, so that each could prevent the other from falling asleep. According to New Zealand army standing orders, the penalty for sleeping on sentry duty in a war zone was death by firing squad. Most people don't know this, and it came as a shock to me when Sgt John Whitworth spelt it out at one of our duty roster briefings. However, the threat of a sudden appearance of the Viet Cong was more of a deterrent for me not to sleep than the fear of execution. I forced myself to stay awake no matter how tired I was. My training with SAS helped in this respect.

Several times during our return patrolling, we came across trails of blood and drag marks. We would follow them for about twenty minutes but would find nothing. Often, we caught the smell of decomposing bodies, but we never found any, as the VC would carefully hide or camouflage their dead. Pigs were plentiful in this area and fed off the corpses. Every time I saw a pig, I felt revolted and gave up eating pork.

Without warning, the front section of 5 Platoon who were leading, came face to face with a lone VC and the lead scout opened fire. We all ran forward and spread out to form a firebase in the usual 'contact front' drill. The VC disappeared but left behind a large blood trail. The front section of 5 Platoon started pursuing him, while the rest of the Company paused for a brief rest.

The lead scout recounted to us the event when they returned.

"The Charlie was easy to follow because he was losing a lot of blood. Being wounded, but able to move, made him very dangerous, so we followed the trail he left carefully. After about 10 minutes, we came across a huge amount of blood where he had stopped and obviously tried to patch himself up, but moved on, probably hearing us approaching. His blood trail was less, but I could still follow him in the thick bush. I tell you; it was real nerve wracking, expecting at any moment for him to ambush us, if he could not keep going.

After another 10 minutes, we came across another huge amount of blood where he was trying to stem its flow. Then nothing. He had moved on and clearly was successful in bounding himself up. Not leaving even a broken branch or footprint that we could follow. He was a damn fine bushman, but damn it, he got away."

As I walked back to my section, I mused at this story and shared in their disappointment. Another body count would make our kill rate ever more impressive. Years later, when I would write this book, and remembered this story, I was then glad he had escaped. I also hoped he had survived the war and lived a full and satisfying life. For truly, he was a real hero. Maybe he even wrote his own book, which I would dearly love to read.

Elements of 274 Regiment were still out there, mauled from the recent fighting but still armed, and dangerous. It was rumoured that they could be moving in our direction. A Bird Dog (spotter plane) had been carefully watching its movements and then it disappeared. High command in Nui Dat was worried that their proximity to V company, then sudden disappearance, could mean that they may be a serious threat to us. I was not able to confirm this, but the following events increased the stakes and our anxiety.

Battalion HQ urged us to move faster towards our LZ, as the enemy force could be battalion size and if they caught up with us, could badly damage if not overrun us. In our present location, there was no cleared area big enough to land helicopters for a company evacuation. To make things worse, our drinking water was nearly all gone. High Command back in Nui Dat considered it was too risky to resupply us for fear of giving our position away. Most of us felt this was not a good reason as the Viet Cong would already know our location, and our strength, most of them being good bushmen, and knowing intimately their own country. Besides, they had a better intelligence system than we did.

Despite all our sophistication with spotter planes (Birddog), starlight scopes, radar, spies, and all the rest of our elaborate intelligence network, we still could not match the enemy. Their intelligence system was the small child playing beside the roadside as we passed; the woodcutter with his oxen cart that passed us on the track, the laundry woman, taxi driver, waiter, the pretty bar girl who seduced servicemen into revealing vital information for the next operation. All Vietnamese in sympathy with the Viet Cong were called into the service against the allies. They were always ahead of us in this area, and one reason they won the war.

The disappearance of 274 Regiment was worrying, especially if they were heading our way. As the enemy traveled with lighter equipment and could move faster intensified all our concerns, as they could show up at any moment.

Moving towards the LZ took many hours moving through thick jungle and difficult terrain that was extremely exhausting. This was made even more challenging, with no water in such hot conditions. Every man was put to the test. As someone later commented, 'If you have a superior enemy force, which is very angry and breathing down your neck, there was no thought about taking a rest no matter how tired you felt.' If Charlie was coming, we knew we had little time to spare. Finally, we made it to the LZ.

Six and a half minutes later (most of us were keeping time) the armada of Huey helicopters were spotted in the distance coming to save us. It was great to be going home to a hot shower and a cold beer. We were all lined up in groups of seven men, being the number for each Huey and standing in our designated pickup positions waiting impatiently.

'Come on you buggers, hurry up!' was the prominent thought of every man standing on that field.

3 minutes later and the air became full of the noise of 25 helicopters all coming in to pick us up … all except ours. The 7 of us stood in horror and disbelief that our Huey had not arrived.

Knowing the standing orders for helicopters, while delivering and extracting troops that staying on the ground for only 5 seconds maximum was because of the danger of enemy snipers. One bullet could easily put a Huey out of action and so it was important to evacuate as quickly as possible, especially in this case.

We looked at each other with a rising fear that they must leave now because they have been on the ground far longer than the designated time and the danger was mounting for the entire company. Each helicopter was bouncing up and down like a wild stallion impatient to leave; demanding to be released, waiting for the order to 'go.' I could see the pilots impatiently looking at watches, red faced with the mounting tension and possible looming disaster.

"Surely to god they won't leave us, will they?" one man whined, trying unsuccessfully to keep the panic out of his voice. We all knew that if we were left, we would all surely die at the hands of the approaching enemy. They rarely took prisoners among non-officers. I could feel my mounting fear and needed all my control not to panic.

The seconds had grown into minutes, and I knew that Major Worsnop would be grappling with the decision to either sacrifice seven of his men for the safety of his whole command or wait for our chopper to arrive. 'Surely, he must give the command to go and leave us behind,' was my strongest thought.

As I stood there in this unfolding drama, I remembered a speech Brian Worsnop made soon after our arrival in Nui Dat. a month earlier.

"I make a promise to every one of you standing here today. My promise to you is that no one will ever be left behind. No one will ever be abandoned to fall into the hands of the enemy. No one!"

'Words are cheap' was one of the comments from some men afterwards. A month later to our current time, his words were being put to the test.

Minutes continued to tick by, and the situation was becoming ever more desperate. Still Maj. Worsnop issued no order to leave.

Now 12 and a half minutes had passed and every man on that field felt this desperation that this could go very badly. Two of our group had dropped their packs and equipment and sat on the ground in resignation. Another angrily shouted out his frustration.

"Were all going to f_cken die. F_ck!"

"I can't believe this," I heard myself whisper, and felt the fear moving up to my throat, making it impossible to speak.

Time kept ticking away. Then out of the swirling dust from the rotor blades of 25 Huey's a co-pilot suddenly appeared in front of us. Our Huey had mistakenly landed at the wrong place at the other end of the field and didn't know where we were.

Him leading the way; we sprinted with all our equipment through the roaring storm of the whirling rotor blades. On arriving, scrambled aboard and immediately the entire armada thundered into the sky, banked sharply to the right as one in perfect formation, straightened out and headed to Nui Dat.

Most of us were so grateful that we were going home safely after a 17-and-a-half-minute certainty that we were going to die on that day. One of the guys angrily questioned the helicopter pilot what happened, yelling over the noise of the Huey. The pilot yelling back over his shoulder; 'profusely apologizing thought that the LZ master had miscalculated the number of men to be picked up in relation to the number of helicopters allocated for the pickup. When our guy asked how such a serious mistake could have been made, when so much was at stake. The pilot replied that such a mistake had happened once before, and so assumed it was a repeat.

"Working it out with operations back in Nui Dat assessed that either you guys were standing in the wrong place or our position in the air fleet was wrong, and all took considerable time," (the longest 17 and a half minutes of my whole life) "to sort out."

A delay that could have ended in tragedy. Even if the rumour of 274 Regiment was not true, the threat of snipers, or even small local VC units attracted by the huge noise of so many helicopters, was very real. They would be able to inflict terrible carnage on such a vulnerable target. At the back of our minds, too, was the fear of not being able to survive on our own. We knew Charlie would arrive at any moment, whether it was elements of 274 or local VC units investigating the commotion.

Whether it was a bad tactical decision by our commanding officer to risk his whole command to save 7 men can be debated and we had luck on our side, but this is not the point. The point is to show how the integrity of one man's word in a leadership role, and his commitment to his team, and that no person is expendable. That every man's safety was his highest priority, which he proved to all of us. Position is what is given, but loyalty and respect cannot be demanded and can only be earned. He certainly earned our undying loyalty and respect on that day. In 2020, I wrote a book called Inspired Leadership, and refer to Maj. Brian Worsnop and his fine leadership.

9

MY NIGHT OF TERROR

To say it was good to be back in Nui Dat and a few days of well-earned rest would be an understatement.

Our tents were pitched in the middle of an abandoned rubber tree plantation, and this caused a problem. Because they had not been bled (harvested) for some years caused them to become top heavy, resulting in some trees falling over without warning. Weighing dangerously heavy, would suddenly snap and come crashing down, destroying anything it fell on. Four of us were engrossed in a game of canasta when we all heard the unmistakable crack right beside our tent. Fortunately, our reflexes were quick, and we were all able to exit before the tree came smashing through the top of our canvas home. We escaped not a moment too soon.

"Bloody hell. If the Viet Cong don't get you, then a bloody rubber tree will!" was one man's summary. Followed by another with:

"So, when informing our families of casualties, they will need to add to the existing WIA, wounded in action, KIA, killed in action, with KBT, killed by bloody tree!" Colin Burgering cut in with his strong English accent and not the slightest hint of the humour being shared.

"That would make it, KBBT."

It probably wasn't all that funny, but as a stress reliever, it was one of the funniest jokes I'd ever heard and responded accordingly, along with the other three guys. An hour later a group of engineers arrived and repaired our home.

Later that day, Alan Haua swapped his SLR (Self-loading rifle) for my M79 grenade launcher and M16 rifle. He wanted to experience the extra firepower for the next operation and be the grenade launcher operative. I was happy for the lighter weight without carrying two weapons and the 15 grenades. He'd checked it out with the boss, Hamish Wilson, beforehand.

I was going to miss the M16 rifle that went with the M79; it was so light with a much lighter bullet and more like a toy compared with the bigger, hard-hitting 7.62mm SLR. No VC was still standing whenever hit with an SLR bullet and they caused horrendous wounds that few ever survived. Most lead scouts opted for the heavier SLR and more reliable weapon. After the exchange, I spent an hour cleaning my new companion. Alan had given it to me in a spotless condition, but in cleaning it brought me into a relationship and a feel for it. I was familiar and trained with SLRs as it was the standard issued weapon in British, New Zealand and Australian Armed Forces in 1968. When I placed it beside my bed that night, it felt more like a close friend that was going to keep me alive during the rest of my tour.

Early on the morning of January 24, 1968, we attended a briefing for 'Operation Coburg', conducted by our new section commander, Paul Hunter. (He was relieving Joe on this 'op'). Paul was a well-built, heavily muscled Māori, and had also served in the SAS.

"Okay, settle down, and listen up, you guys. We are being moved by choppers to the border area between Ben Hoa and Long Khanh Province. Bien Hoa is where the big Yank air base is, and we are going by Huey's later this morning. For those of you who don't know, Bien Hoa is about eighty miles away northwest of here. There's three hardcore NVA regiments and a large VC Rocket regiment that have been spotted in the area. The Yanks are worried they may try to take the air base out, or at least blast hell out of it with their rockets. Our job is to stop them if they try or find them first and destroy them. Most of the Aussie task force will be involved, and several Yank infantry units are also on their way to reinforce the air base. This Op's going to make Duntroon look like a picnic, so I'm told by Company Headquarters. So, get a good breakfast. No one knows when we'll eat fresh food again."

"Bugger me, Paul. Eating bloody ration packs for more than three days is like eating shit," one man complained.

"Well, the way you make those bloody curries, I thought you already were," someone sniggered, and a chuckle went round the gathered men. I looked around at them. We always referred to ourselves as 'the boys', and when we had arrived two months earlier, we had been so young and fresh-faced; now a hardened and haggard look was beginning to show.

"By the way, guys," Paul continued.

"This is Gunner Ellwood from 161 (New Zealand artillery battery stationed in Nui Dat) and he will be joining us as a forward artillery observer, and I want one of you guys to look after him. Say, you Sas. Can you keep an eye on him?"

"Sure, Paul, I can do that." I answered.

After the briefing, I wandered over to where Ellwood was sitting, separate from the rest of the Platoon.

"Hi, I'm Sisson, but most of us have nicknames here and mine's Sas."

He jumped to his feet. Gidday, I'm Ellwood, Stuart is my first and nick name, I guess." We shook hands, and I instantly liked him.

"Where are you from?" I asked.

"Foxton."

"Really? I'm from just down the road from you, in Levin." I retorted.

"Oh, you're the guys who don't know how to play rugby." He jokingly mocked.

"Well, I remember when I was in 3rd grade and our team thrashed the daylights out of you guys. I think we all agreed afterwards that we would give Foxton a 20-point lead at the start of the next game just to make it interesting for us."

We both laughed at the hilarity of our conversation and felt that instant bond. It always amazed me that typical New Zealand humour often involved good natured mockery and even insults as a way of sharing friendship.

By 8.00 am, we moved with the rest of the company towards the airfield, where our choppers were waiting to fly us towards Bien Hoa. It was already getting hot, and I could feel the sweat trickling down the centre of my back, dampening my shirt, not only from the heat and also from some nervousness, sensing some awaited danger. The road was lined with hundreds of trucks and APCs (Armoured Personnel Carriers) all filled with Australian troops waiting for their orders to move out. Red dust was kicked up by the passing vehicles, as well as by Centurion tanks, mounted with their big 105mm guns. They were all heading for Ben Hoa. This was the biggest concentration of troops and firepower I'd ever seen. Clearly, this operation really means business.

An hour later, V. Company lifted off in our armada of helicopters and within thirty minutes flew over Fire Base Anderson, which was close to the operational area we were to be landed.

Fire bases were defensive positions, usually held by an infantry company protecting one or two 105mm artillery batteries and heavy mortars. They were surrounded by fortifications, barbed wire, minefields, and bunkers. Fire bases were numerously spread out over most of South Vietnam, allowing the allies to cover most of the country in quick response and rapid artillery fire to support infantry units in contact with enemy forces. Not surprisingly, we felt that there was no way the Viet Cong could ever win this war.

As our chopper, in unison with the air armada, came roaring in to land, each man was readying himself to leap from their Huey and run for cover. Even though we were coming into a safe area unlike the last operation, there was always the threat of snipers lying in wait to take a man out before dissolving back into the cover of the jungle.

As the man in front of me leaped from the Huey, his lightweight tent fell out of his pack. I scooped down to pick it up, knowing he would need it, but as I straightened up to pass through the open door, my rifle barrel hit the top of the chopper doorway and forcefully bounced back, and the rifle sights struck into my head with such a blow that it knocked me flat on my back. Two Australian helicopter crew (the two side machine gunners) picked me up and threw me out of the door so that I landed on my feet, running. The Huey immediately took off, and I staggered like a drunkard, dizzy, my head swimming and throbbing with pain. I could barely see as a more than usual amount of sweat was running into my eyes.

"Sniper, get down," I heard someone quite close to me yell.

"My God, find cover quick. VC snipers rarely miss," they had warned us. I threw myself down behind a small bush that afforded little protection, but at least some cover from a sniper's view.

I lay there dazed and struggled to stay conscious. I couldn't afford to pass out. Then, from nowhere, a medic appeared beside me.

"Where are you hit, man?"

"I'm not hit, I just …" As I spoke, I looked down to see the front of my shirt covered in blood.

"Fuckin' hell, I am hit," I blurted out. "Shit. Where am I hit? Where am I hit?" I was in a panic as I frantically felt all over my chest and stomach. It was commonly known that serious and fatal wounds were often not felt by the victim. When I broke my arm playing rugby years before, it had been several minutes before I felt any pain. I couldn't find the wound, and I was becoming hysterical, as there was so much blood.

"Bugger me, you've been shot in the head," the medic suddenly said. My hand touched the area where I'd been hit with my rifle sights. It came away covered in blood and was oozing out of the wound in incredible amounts just above the hairline. I remembered from my army first aid training that head wounds bleed excessively heavily, even from a slight scratch, and was very relieved that I hadn't been shot. I figured out that as they had thrown me from the chopper, someone had seen me running with blood streaming, and had concluded that a sniper had shot me. The medic put in three stitches, dressed the wound, removed most of the blood from my face with a wet cloth and left me. I changed my shirt and discarded the blood soaked one under a bush, just as Blue Neame came over to me.

"You okay Sas?"

"Yeah. It's just a scratch. I'm fine." I sounded tough, but it was only to cover the strong nausea I was feeling.

Stuart appeared and sat down beside me. "Shit, you look a mess. Are you alright?" I nodded and Stuart continued. "You can't meet Charlie with such a dirty face." He poured some water on a rag and wiped the remaining caked blood from my face. His caring friendship touched me.

"Yeah, I just whacked my head on my rifle sights as I exited the chopper and I have a thumping headache. I feel a bit like throwing up, but I'll be fine."

Stuart looked at my discarded bloodied shirt lying under the small bush, "Wow, look at your shirt. You must have lost a lot of blood. You look a little pale. I'll carry your pack if you like."

"No, I'm all good, and I think we are being signalled to move out. Let's go."

We moved several hundred metres and formed a harbour. There I lit a cigarette, fighting hard not to vomit. Soon after, the company moved off, heading east, passing through some very thick bamboo that cut our clothes to ribbons and flesh if you mistakenly grabbed hold of it. It took us most of the day to travel only fifteen hundred metres and then camped up for the night. My head throbbed throughout the day, making it difficult to concentrate and stay alert. There were many enemy signs, and it was essential for every man to keep his wits about him.

The next morning my head felt a little better, but I still felt nauseous, and skipped preparing myself breakfast, settling for just a cup of tea.

Stuart's shell scrape was next to mine, and I briefly passed to him some tactics of infantry troops in a defensive position. Being a gunner in the artillery, this was new for him. I also told him to speak only whispering, as talking normally carried quite a distance through the jungle and could give our position away to any possible unwelcomed listeners. He attempted to hold friendly conversations with me throughout the day, but I felt too sick to respond to his friendliness and regretted this as we enjoyed each other's company.

An hour later, Six Platoon moved to a new area 500 metres away to set up an ambush on a track junction. While I was digging my shell scrape, I dug up a huge tarantula that landed on my boot. I nearly fainted with fright, and instinctively reacted by sending it to the next world with my shovel.

It was a quiet night and the next morning I could eat something as my nausea was a little less. We moved out early. One section leading, and two section (us) bringing up the rear. Soon after, our departure shots rang out up front.

"Contact front!" came the yell from the front section. As we ran forward preparing to fan out to form a wide front and return fire, the usual enemy contact drill, we passed through a large clearing. Without warning, a VC to our left only thirty metres away opened fire on us with an AK47 automatic weapon. Fortunately for us, he was firing wildly, probably in panic at our sudden appearance, and bullets kicked up the ground around and thudded into the trees behind us. I quickly noticed that we were bunched up, Stuart being right beside me, a perfect target for the VC. I signalled with my free arm to him to spread out. With hearts pumping wildly, we all scattered and managed to safely find cover and returned fire. The VC disappeared and escaped. Within seconds, shells came roaring in, tearing up the area 150 metres away. Our gunners were more accurate this time, including a greater safety zone between us and the falling shells.

One Section had killed two VC in the skirmish and suffered no losses. Barney Tautau had been the lead scout and was one of the best in the company. Lt. Wilson ordered One Section to take up the rear of the platoon, while our section took over the lead. As I walked past Barney, I noticed he was very pale, unusually so for a Māori.

"Well done, Barney," I murmured, then stopped in my tracks, by the gruesome sight of two bodies lying on the ground before me. One VC had taken a bullet between his eyes and it had split his head right down the middle, his brains having been splattered over a nearby bush. I looked down at them, feeling neither compassion nor hate. I wasn't even revolted at the sight, but simply felt numb. In that moment, I knew that my humanity was sliding away as I hardened to all this ugliness. Then, for a brief moment, it returned as I felt sorry for their families, who would soon learn that their sons had died this day. I thought of my family in New Zealand, and how they would react if they were to learn about my death.

Walking past the dead, I noticed that the second one was lying on his back, mouth wide open. His teeth were filled with gold. It was a popular Asian custom to have most of one's teeth capped with their personal wealth to offset their old age.

'He's not going to need that anymore,' I thought grimly. Smashing my rifle butt into his mouth caused his whole face and upper jaw to cave in from a massive bullet exit hole in the back of his head. I leaned against a tree and spewed up what little food I had in my stomach.

"Haven't the guts for it, eh, Sas?" I heard someone laugh behind me.

"He can keep his bloody gold," I spat out as I walked on, disgusted at what I was becoming.

We moved on, and an hour later, the 'thumbs down' signal (the enemy is sighted, message) was passed. down the line of men from our lead scouts. Two VC had been spotted in the distance, but they were too far away to engage and then disappeared. We sighted nothing else for the rest of our patrol and stopped later in the afternoon to set up an ambush.

I was starting to suffer from acute diarrhoea. I'd eaten hardly anything throughout the day and couldn't face an evening meal from the ration pack. I looked apathetically at a tin of beef and threw it back into my pack.

"I'll do your shift in the ambush so you can have a good night's rest."

"Thanks Stuart, but no. I'll be okay. You need your rest just as much." His caring gesture again touched me.

After relieving myself for the third time in the last 3 hours, I rolled up on the ground and managed a few hours' sleep before it was my turn to man the ambush.

The next morning, the 27th, we set off by crossing a river and early in the afternoon, linked up with the rest of the company. We were resupplied with water and rations by helicopters. My stomach felt a little better, but it could only tolerate tinned fruit and dried biscuits.

Throughout the day, there was a constant sound of fighting in the distance, mingled with shell fire. Reports coming in mentioned that 8 Australians had been killed, with many more wounded. With many fresh signs of the enemy in this area, there was a sense of foreboding that something was building up to some climatic event. A happening that would change the lives of the entire population of South Vietnam. The Communist Tet Offensive was about to take place.

High Command also sensed something was about to happen and ordered all platoons to re-join their companies for extra safety. In mid-afternoon we moved to a new location at company strength, and for the next two hours waded through swamp, thick with leeches and Goodness knows what else. 'May this be the last swamp I ever see,' was my fervent thought.

That night, three section did not adhere to standard procedure of putting up a perimeter vine, or a piece of string around their part of the platoon harbour. This perimeter vine enabled sentries to find their way to and from the ambush site without losing their way in the dark. As it was a dark night with no moon, it took Alan Haua and me over an hour after our sentry duties to find our bed spaces. Losing precious sleep through such neglect merely placed an extra burden on our already overtaxed bodies and minds. I felt angry at members of 3 section, but was even more frightened by the thought that we may have wandered off into the jungle and become permanently lost in the nearby swamp. It took me another hour to drop off to sleep, so stirred up was my mind.

The next day, we headed out of the swamp area, much to everyone's relief. At midday, we had another 'contact front' with the enemy. Two VC killed, with no loss to ourselves.

"You okay, Stuart?" I asked at the next rest break.

"Yeah, but I will be as glad as hell to get back to my unit and be cosy in Firebase Anderson or Nui Dat. I'm over this bloody 'grunt.' (Infantry soldier) patrolling. I'm leaving 6 Platoon tomorrow and will be with Company HQ for the rest of the op." (operation).

"Stay in touch when you get back to 161. Let's have a beer or two between operations." I suggested. He nodded his agreement.

In mid-afternoon, firing broke out to our rear, followed by explosions. Because of the density of the jungle, we had passed an enemy patrol, only two or three metres away without seeing each other. Minutes later, they bumped into our Company HQ section, further down the line, where they saw each other at the same time. The enemy was quicker to react, and one fired an RPG rocket launcher, barely missing two signalmen before being cut down in a hail of bullets. Another, although shot several times by M16 bullets (clearly not from an SLR) threw a large anti-tank grenade that exploded on impact. The next volley of fire from our guys blew his brains out, and he died with a second grenade still in his hand. Two of HQ section were wounded. The rest of the enemy patrol escaped. Sergeant-Major Hayward had a hard time retrieving the unexploded grenade from the hand of the dead VC. By securing it with string and pulling it from a distance finally set it off with a loud explosion.

There was little left of the dead enemy soldier. The HQ section captured several RPGs, large amounts of explosives, ammunition, drugs, money and six packs, showing the number in their patrol.

The job of searching the dead and their kits was given to me and the company Intelligence non-commissioned officer (IO). While searching them, I noticed they were wearing the green uniforms of North Vietnamese regulars (NVA). These were better trained and more highly motivated soldiers, compared to the VC irregulars we had mainly met, and they had certainly died bravely enough.

It was not pleasant searching them, as they were badly mutilated and disfigured from their gunshot deaths. A crazy thought that was to repeat itself every day for the rest of my tour and beyond, was: 'If I'm killed, I hope that I'm spared looking like this. A quick clean shot through the heart will do. Please, not through the face or head, like these poor bastards. Hell, war is ugly.'

I reached into the breast pocket of the one I was searching, pulled out a wallet and opened it. A black-and-white photograph fell out onto the ground. I picked it up, and saw the man's family – a young wife, and two small children, a boy, and a girl, looking at me, smiling. I choked.

"Bloody hell, look at this." I handed it to the IO. He looked at it, shrugged with no expression on his face, and handed it back to me. I carefully put the photo back into the wallet and respectfully slipped it back into the dead man's pocket. Afterwards, I walked back to the platoon position feeling numb, again not knowing how to feel, and questioning how I had put myself in to this crazy war.

On my return, I could not find Stuart and learned that he was in a meeting with Company HQ. I discovered there were no acceptable sleeping spots left within the perimeter of our section, and finally found one five metres outside the perimeter vine. It was a decision I was to regret. After struggling to dig my shell scrape with such low energy, and then was able to down a light meal and a cup of tea, at the protest of still a delicate stomach, it was my turn on sentry, from 6 to 8 pm. I was thankful that they had given me the easiest shift and was looking forward to a good night's sleep afterwards. Returning to my shell scrape from sentry duty, my stomach was constantly rumbling painfully. Sleep Wouldn't come.

After several hours, I drifted into crazy dreams of madness and was surrounded by little red demons all reaching out and clutching my legs, competing for my attention. Suddenly, I was jolted awake by a real demon with the most blood-curdling scream, only metres away from me in the darkness. I sat bolt upright, clutching my rifle, frozen in terror. I vividly imagined what might have caused such a horrific cry. Remembering the two mangled NVA soldiers we'd searched, that were about 60 metres away where we had left them. The cry must have been from pigs, eating the corpses, I reasoned. Slowly lowering myself into the prone position, I agonised over them being consumed in such a way.

The mind plays strange tricks when frozen in fear. In my befuddled state, I imagined the NVA soldier with the photograph was still alive and being, 'oh my god', eaten alive by wild pigs, and agonised further at his painful and lingering death. The scream in the night was no doubt from a pig, but I was sure it had come from him. Then I imagined he craved revenge against me personally for violating him by searching through his personal things. My mind twisted this further by imagining that, while he was still being eaten, crawled in my direction to kill me with his bayonet clenched between his teeth. I really believed this. I wanted to get up and run, run anywhere, but away from my self-consumed insanity. I found I was powerless to move, powerless to even reach for my rifle beside me to defend myself against him, as he, in agony, dragged the pigs along as they consumed him through the undergrowth to cut my throat. How long I lay there agonizing with my mind rapidly disintegrating, I will never know.

Suddenly, only one metre from my head, I heard him with a rustle of leaves and the snap of a twig. This was not my imagination. I sensed something, or someone, almost close enough to touch. I was totally paralysed with fear. I couldn't breathe. My wounded, pain-crazed enemy had found me. This was my end. 'Oh, my God, what a way to die,' was my only thought. Seconds passed. I felt as if barbed wire were being dragged through my intestines and stomach. I could still hear the slight movements of my executioner as he moved ever so slowly towards me, sniffing the air. As I resigned myself to die something finally snapped inside me. My head rolled to one side and a muffled moan escaped my lips. With that, there was a scurrying sound as a pig bolted off into the darkness.

I shook all over and fought back the tears screaming to be released. Even though part of my mind worked out that it was probably the pig that had uttered the blood-curdling scream that caused me so much terror, yet another part of me still believed that only a miracle had saved me from the revengeful, wounded NVA. I finally fell asleep around 4am. Two hours later, I was woken to 'stand to'.

Afterwards Stuart found me and told me that as he was going to be with Company HQ for the rest of the operation that I could have his shell scrape inside the platoon perimeter. I was too embarrassed to tell him of my traumatising night experience. I was sad to see him go and would miss his cheerful nature. At least he will be safer with HQ section than with us, the equivalent of being on the front line.

I was feeling ill and had to relieve myself about three times every hour. The good news was that the Vietnamese Tet holiday was starting the next day. During this time, both sides of the conflict had decided on a truce. I was more than thankful that I would finally get some rest, so I thought. Little did any of us know that the largest battle of the entire war was about to explode.

10
KATHRYN

I started breathing as Margaret, my Breath Integration practitioner, directed. After about 10 minutes, I felt deep feelings stirring. I knew that the breath was taking me into a deep, dark, and painful place in my past that I really didn't want to go. Then, without warning, I could smell cordite as if firecrackers had been let off in the room. The association of dead and broken bodies filled my mind, along with confusion, fear, and dread about what was surfacing.

"I can't do this, Maggie."

"There is nothing you have to do. Just feel."

"These feelings are too much. I can't go there. You don't understand." I desperately whispered back.

"We don't have to understand what's coming up. Don't try to understand anything. Just feel the energy in your body to what the breath is bringing up."

I'd had many sessions before this, which had dealt with many other less painful aspects of my life, mostly from childhood. But now, something new was stirring. As I continued to breathe, I felt the dreaded memories and feelings from Vietnam coming and I really didn't want to feel them. It felt like being re-traumatised by the past suppressed feelings all over again. My experience with this method had clearly shown me that one is never re-traumatized by facing the past in this conscious way. In fact, trying to escape and bury our feelings is a bigger contributor to being traumatized. That the only real way of releasing the pain was to feel it. If we can't feel it, then we can feel our resistance to feeling it. This is the resistance to feeling my emotions and wanting to escape, avoid, or deny. Knowing all this, a part of me was still wanting to pretend that everything was good or positive, but I knew it was not. I could feel the tightness in my body, mostly in the solar plexus, and knew that by putting my full attention there where the strongest physical sensation was would release it, but I was so afraid to do this simple thing and free myself.

The memory of a VC suddenly appearing only 30 metres away and firing automatic fire at us while bunched up and in the open came flooding back. My fear for Stuart's safety and my other comrades, Blue, Graham and Alan, and for myself. Then my memory shifted to a dead VC laying on his back, mouth wide open and his gold-laden teeth sparkling in the sunlight and the disgust in myself in what followed. My mind shifted again to me laying in the night, totally petrified as I imagined a revengeful North Vietnamese soldier, his bayonet between his teeth crawling towards me, to cut my throat. The image in my mind was made more terrifying with the horror of him being consumed by wild pigs as he crawled towards me. All those images. Memories and the feelings associated were with me again after all these years. This showed that I was still carrying that traumatic burden. Until it was released, I would continue to carry that pain that would influence every area of my life, every decision, and every experience. That painful event was staring me in the face, inviting me to face and release it. I took a deeper breath and let myself fall into the abyss of the unknown.

With each passing second, the memories grew stronger as they unfolded, a multitude of feelings in conflict with each other lying beneath the mental/emotional surface. I could feel my resistance to feeling them and my body began to twist, as muscles tensed in an attempt to escape what was coming up.

I could hear Maggie, yet her voice seemed a million miles away, gently speaking to feel these feelings. Her voice was soothing, inviting me to trust the healing process. Minutes passed as I struggled with these memories. Part of me wanting to feel them, and another part desperately striving to control what I was feeling. I was locked in an internal battle that I could not surrender to. While struggling and sobbing with frustration and fear, my clothes became drenched in sweat as my body heaved and twisted in an effort to escape. Her comforting voice enabled me to re-focus on what was happening inside of me, rather than be lost in the memories.

I switched my mind from the memory images back into my emotions and into my body, and that was violently shaking. Holding my attention there, I began to be fully present with it.

Without warning, the miracle happened. As intense as the pain, fear, and dread had been, they were suddenly all gone. I felt a deep peace as the trauma had been integrated and released. My feelings of terror only seconds ago were replaced by a deep love. Not a love for a person or thing, but a love for its own sake. It was so strong and overwhelming in its beauty that I could not contain it and gently wept as part of the release. My body felt so relaxed. The shaking was gone. These overwhelming beautiful feelings were the same I'd felt in Vietnam, when everything slowed down during my worst moments that I had then mistakenly associated with insanity. I could sense Maggie's presence and hear her gently whispering how magnificent I had done.

Afterwards, with a cup of tea, we gently talked as Margaret praised me for my willingness to face the past and become free of it.

"You certainly are a fighter." She commented. "It is so amazing how every person responds differently to this process. Some struggle, like you, others escape into sleep or distracting behaviour, while others simply freeze. The fight/flight/freeze syndrome that all humans have. But every time each person eventually reaches that integration and releases the trauma."

I simply nodded, recognizing this most truly miraculous process of simply breathing and being fully present with what I felt was enough to release such past trauma. No drugs, no therapy, not even having to talk about it was all it took. One day, perhaps psychotherapy will discover this amazingly simple process of presence. It is truly the most important thing I have ever learned in my whole life.

Most sessions are rarely as intense as the one I just had, being very gentle and yet just as powerful. The reason this one was so intense was because of my resistance to feel my feelings. The more we resist, the more intense it becomes. Knowing that, strugglers like me have the added inconvenience of making the sessions longer and less comfortable. But we get there in the end as soon as we put our full attention on the resistance in the body. But, at last I was feeling, whereas since Vietnam I had refused to feel anything less than positive, which would account for my poor health.

Remembering what my psychology professor said at one of his lectures when I studied psychology years earlier came to mind.

"The sickest people in our community are those that have a lot of stress, a lot of buried trauma, but feel nothing." I remembered back then how I had nodded with enthusiastic agreement, not imagining for a second that he was talking about people like me, despite my neurotic behaviour. In the words of Carl Jung, one of the founding fathers of modern psychology, when he said:

"Neurosis is always a substitute for legitimate suffering." In other words, we need to have the courage to face our fears; face our pain and deal with our problems. Yet, the substitute, the avoidance or escapist behaviour, the neurosis itself becomes a bigger problem than what people are trying to escape from. People will try to escape this pain and so build layer on top of layer or more neurosis. You can clearly see this in alcoholics, drug addicts, in all mental, emotional, and physical addictions, phobias, and this perfectly described me.

Yes, it takes all our courage to do this. The alternative is to deny, avoid, distract ourselves, and hope that it all goes away. The problem with this approach is that feelings buried alive never die and come back to haunt us later in life as mental illness, neurosis, and physical disease.

The bottom line is that there is no escape from suppressed trauma. One day we are all going to meet it, either through facing it head on (what I recommend perhaps in a process like Breath Integration, or holistic psychology) or we will meet it when in a crisis, such as a marriage breakup, bankruptcy, failing health, and mental decline. Yet even in this 11th hour, we can still meet it if we are conscious of what we feel about the current crisis. This is often enough to release it forever and many people that have been traumatised have made this discovery. But the first option of meeting the pain head-on is easier, even though it seems like it is not.

This was the sixth session with Margaret, and she was an excellent Breath Integration Practitioner, allowing me to feel safe with my own feelings. I felt secure, allowing myself to be this vulnerable with her.

Sitting there feeling at peace with myself, fresh memories were stirring, those of more recent events. The hurt I felt from my break-up with Rita felt resolved from an earlier session. All that remained was a beautiful feeling of love for her. Now a different memory was coming up in my mind from 5 years before, of Kathryn.

Eighteen months after my marriage break-up with Rita, I had left my job and moved to a yoga centre called Aio Wira, in the Waitakere ranges close to Auckland. I'd had it with women, with jobs, with careers, with life. I wanted to escape everything. Taking a vow of celibacy, I lived like a monk, while throwing myself completely into my studies. This year at Aio Wira, even though it was an escape from life, was a wonderful time of personal exploration. It introduced me to many new ideas: yoga, meditation, Hindu philosophy, Buddhism, Taoism, while keeping my studies of the Qabalah with Michael Freedman.

I kept my academic studies going at night school, covering economics, business law and psychology. This I found very balancing, one left brain and the other right brain gave me an interesting balance between feminine and masculine aspects of myself. It was good fortune and not by any intelligent design on my part that I had embarked on these pursuits.

I experimented a lot with breathing and developed several supporting processes that brought me closer to the present moment through expanding awareness. I was trying to recreate those amazing experiences in Vietnam when everything slowed down, and where I felt completely at peace and in love with life. My experimenting and research brought me close, but not quite and years later I would discover that you cannot reach for being here and now as a striving, as this is still aiming for a better future, which blocks the experience of the elusive present 'now.' I was to later recognise that in the present moment, there is no striving, no aiming points, no fear, no beliefs, no philosophies, no techniques. Just pure experience!

It was at Aio Wira that I started my first book, called: *Rebirthing Made Easy*. This was my first attempt at expressing the many new ideas and inspirations that were forming in me. It was a poorly written account of my work, full of misguided positive thinking concepts I had learned that had more to do with suppressing actual feelings than truly expanding awareness. But when it was published two years later, it became an international success, much to my surprise.

I'd also started to teach both meditation and the breathing technique, rebirthing, and had several students. I continued with the Gurdjieff work and the Qabalah. Colour healing caught my attention for a while, but it was breathwork that held centre stage for me, and was the closest thing I'd come across that enabled me to feel safe enough to feel my feelings. Feeling my emotions was something I'd spent most of my life avoiding, especially since Vietnam. I had always believed, as most people do, that the emotions harboured all one's pain. But breathwork led me to discover that the intellectual mind was the storehouse of our sufferings and that feelings were the innocent expression of that pain or dread. And when felt while being fully present with them, released the emotional and mental anguish from the mind and the body.

This revelation was the most inspirational experience of my inner exploration. It became the basis of many books to follow over the coming 40 years, notably, 'The Truth of Your Moment', probably being the most important, co-authored with Magdalena Janicka and published in 2020.

It was 1984, and I'd been involved with extensive inner work for over four years, but still had a lot more exploration ahead of me. Most

Breath Integration sessions revolved around daily irritations, self-esteem issues, and such like. A few memories of Vietnam that had surfaced had been released. Nothing major, though, that led me to conclude that I was now clear of trauma from the war. Yet I still became upset whenever I was asked about my time there, or any discussion about Vietnam. I suspected there was still a lot of suppressed and unconscious fear still inside of me I didn't want to face. Not until I started working with Margaret 5 years later when the full force of suppressed terror from the worst moments of my life emerged and made themselves known.

After a year at Aio Wira, I felt I was nearly ready to move back to the city and back into life again.

One afternoon, I stood at the window of the centre main hall and outside on the lawn was a woman with her back to me, talking to Ray, another Aio Wira resident. 'There's my future wife,' was the thought that immediately shot through my mind. I quickly dismissed it as another trick of my ego that was by now struggling with my celibacy. I turned away, telling myself that I was not yet ready to let go of that safety valve. Ray then walked into the hall, followed by a woman who I thought was probably the most beautiful I had ever seen.

Her name was Kate and was Australian. She had recently arrived with her New Zealand boyfriend and was interested in learning yoga and meditation.

I agreed that I'd teach her meditation. For the next four months, we worked together, including breathing sessions. I liked Kate, and we felt safe with each other, her already being in a relationship. This situation changed a little when her relationship broke up, but we continued working together just as good friends.

After leaving Aio Wira and moving down from the hills into Auckland, Kate and I still saw each other once a week for sessions and friendship, but nothing more. I felt her name, Kate, sounded too harsh and asked her if she would mind me calling her Kathryn, which in my mind more suited her. She agreed, and this seemed to signal to being emotionally closer, though I told myself that I was still not ready to have an intimate relationship.

About this time, I met a lovely woman, Theresa, with whom I couldn't avoid having a beautiful romance. In this, I discovered I was still afraid of the closeness Theresa offered. Despite my fear, I was approaching some readiness to come back into the mainstream of life. However, Theresa was so caring and lovely and therefore too much of a threat to my fear of intimacy and so ended the brief relationship with her. I had no awareness that my buried wounds would be exposed by love as they had been with

Rita. This exposure of pain would have been too much to cope with, even though it would have led to my healing. Thus, I falsely concluded that we were not compatible with each other and walked away from love and a major healing opportunity.

Kathryn was such a joy to be with in our sessions together. My pain from Vietnam slid even more into suppression, as all trauma does when everything in life is going well. It was later when life challenges happened, did the pain surface again.

Kathryn had such a gentle nature. Experiencing her closeness in our sessions together, while keeping her at arm's length, physically made her safe. Then, one day during one of her weekly sessions, I noticed that something was troubling her. When I questioned her about what I was observing, she revealed she was going back to Australia in two weeks. An old friend had contacted her and offered her a good position in his company in Melbourne. She had accepted it.

Suddenly, the bottom of my world caved in. She would leave my life forever. At that moment, she became vitally important to me. You never know the value of things and especially people until you are about to lose them. Choking back the tears, I asked her if she could stay an extra two weeks to complete her training with me as a practitioner in the Breath Integration process. She agreed and would change her air tickets to accommodate this.

We held each other's gaze, and I noticed a tear in the corner of her eye and no doubt she noticed mine. Her agreement to stay longer gave us four weeks to complete our work together and, for me, precious time for what I had in mind. Two weeks later I proposed marriage to her, and a week after that, gave me her answer. We were married a year later.

As I look over my life, it has been far from elegant or graceful, full of mistakes. But with women, I have been truly blessed. When we enter an intimate relationship with someone, we are influenced by the other person, positively and negatively. There is no avoiding this. We unconsciously change to accommodate our partner. But, for my good fortune, I hit the jackpot every time. Rita had seen me through my nightmares, allowing me to function in everyday affairs and essentially had given me back my life through her love. Kathryn lifted me to a new level of believing in myself, which reflected in success in most things I went into. She believed in me more than I did and more than she did in herself. She saw my potential and continually encouraged me to take the next step.

Over the next five years, I wrote three books and became a successful international speaker and breathwork trainer. Together, we were dynamic. Kathryn's gentle, open nature made her a wonderful partner in the sensitive counselling work we were doing.

Despite our success, we had some difficulties along the way. Some close friends and colleagues in the Rebirthing community turned against me after the release of my first book, *Rebirthing Made Easy*. I felt hurt and disappointed at their reaction and to this day; I have never fully understood why. Kathryn had, as usual, some wise, comforting and thought-provoking advice to give me.

"They may be jealous of your success, and probably have something to learn from this. Watching your reaction, you probably do, as well. But don't let their actions make you small. You're only as big as what it takes to upset you. I know you are bigger than this."

Despite my success, at a deep level, a battle still raged within me from the legacy of the war. A battle that projected a struggle into everyday life. These became activated with big and small irritating confrontations with life events. My conflict with the Rebirthing association was just one of those projections.

After two years together, we had a son, David. who inherited her good looks and gentle nature, which won him some TV show acting roles in his future. He was a sensitive child, and I was better prepared for a parental role than from my first two girls.

Kathryn was a wonderful mother, and her focus changed from business partner to motherhood. Suddenly, my main partner could not be totally there for me as she had been. Her energy was now rightfully needed elsewhere, but the unhealed child in me felt neglected. To compensate, I flung myself deeper into my work, running several companies and more writing (my usual way of avoiding life issues). We exchanged our small two bedroomed house for a much larger five-bedroom property in a more desirable part of Auckland. Success continued to follow me, but the marriage was beginning to falter. Once again, I was falling yet again into distracting behaviour to cope.

Around this time, Vietnam's memories surfaced. How easily I would fall into combat mode, which showed itself in uncontrollable anger fits. I would break things, yell, become abusive, but fortunately I never attacked or directed my venom against anyone physically. Just situations that I was not coping with.

I felt more defensive and withdrawn. My trainings, counselling work and business dealings still flourished, but financial profits were dropping.

In February 1991, Kathryn and I mutually agreed to separate. Once again, I walked away from love, unconsciously threatened by it, that could upset my status quo. But we parted as genuine friends, which reflected our whole relationship. Even at the lowest point of our marriage, we never stopped loving each other. Her generous nature and our connection with David have ensured that we remained emotionally close to this day.

Through the many sessions I'd had, my emotions were freeing up. This meant that buried traumas were more easily coming to the surface, and this was such a vital part of the healing process. But it was still slow going, and it wasn't for another 15 years of experimenting and refining it that sped up the healing process to today's highly efficient method. This was thanks to the many people who would come into my life, mainly Marina Kitchatova from Russia and Magdalena Janicka from Poland, who co-founded the latest development, which became titled Integrative Presence.

But in 1991, knowing I still had much healing still to do, was when I reached out to Margaret to have breath integration sessions with. With Margaret's help, she could allow me to see the connection between what was happening with me and Kathryn and the pain still in me from Vietnam. Over a series of sessions, the ancient memories of those terrible days surfaced I had carefully blanked out as not to feel.

Margaret kept reminding me of my own teachings that these need to come up and be faced if they are to be integrated and released.

These sessions helped me through the current crisis to get my life back into focus, but predictably, it brought up many new memories for me to deal with from my darkest days.

11
THE TET OFFENSIVE

The company had moved 600 metres from its former position and dug in, in the usual all-round defensive harbour. We were to wait until the end of the Tet holiday, and then try to find the 274 VC regiment and the NVA units operating in this area.

It was January 29th, 1968, and Vietnam was about to be shattered by the largest communist offensive of the entire war. Assembled throughout South Vietnam were 80,000 Viet Cong and North Vietnamese main-line troops, poised for a single thrust to take over the entire south and win the war. Supporting them were many thousands more regional Viet Cong units carefully prepared for the coming battle. The prelude to this offensive was the siege of Khesanh.

KHESANH

General Giap, commanding the Communist forces in the war, seemed not to have been discouraged by his troop losses throughout his build-up to the Tet offensive. His initial target of the Tet Offensive was the American base at Khesanh, twenty kilometres south of the DMZ (Demilitarized Zone), near the Laotian border. General Westmoreland, the allied commander, had intended the base at Khesanh to be a staging area for operations into Laos against the Ho Chi Minh trail. However, these operations were never put into effect from this base after the coming storm.

When US intelligence revealed a massive NVA build-up in the area that amounted to four divisions, as well as many artillery batteries and one armoured unit, 40,000 troops, Westmoreland despatched heavy reinforcements to Khesanh.

As both sides prepared for a showdown, the memory of Dien Bien

Phu was on everyone's mind. The battle of Dien Bien Phu, 15 years earlier, when Giap besieged an isolated French garrison and eventually destroyed it was the decisive and final military victory over the French.

The siege of Khesanh, from January 20 to April 6, 1968, produced appalling losses on both sides, particularly for the Communists. About 10,000 NVA soldiers and over 500 Americans were killed. Most of the slaughter of the enemy was the work of American B-52 air strikes.

The Allies were convinced that Khesanh was the real target of the Offensive, and that the widespread Tet operations were mainly a diversion. After the war, the Communists insisted Khesanh was the diversion for Tet that proved to be successful, despite its huge losses. It was successful because it drew large numbers of American units away from the many key targets, leaving them open to the main offensive. Historians are still debating whether the siege at Khesanh was a successful feint or a strategic disaster for Giap.

THE TET OFFENSIVE

The Communist attacks in the border regions, including Khesanh, were to prepare for the main assault throughout the entire country, scheduled to begin on the first day of Tet – the sacred celebration of the Lunar New Year. Each year both sides had traditionally honoured a ceasefire, and so the timing was planned to catch the allies by surprise. It was also scheduled because it was the anniversary of the legendary Tet victory in 1789, when the Vietnamese defeated the Chinese in the battle of Hanoi. On the eve of the offensive, Radio Hanoi broadcast a poem written by Ho Chi Minh:

"This spring far outshines all previous springs, / Of victories throughout the land come happy. tidings. / Let north and south emulate each other in fighting the United States' aggressors! / Forward! Total victory will be ours!'"

On the early morning of January 30th, the Tet campaign erupted, with attacks on the nine largest cities and thirty provincial capitals, with the main thrust on Saigon, and Hue, the ancient city in the north of the country. If Hue, close to the well-infiltrated DMZ, could be captured, it would be relatively easy to be reinforced with fresh NVA troops from North Vietnam. If Saigon could be taken and held, the psychological effect would be immense, hopefully leading to the Americans suing for peace.

During the weeks leading up to the attack, 4000 VC infiltrated Saigon, dressed as farmers, vegetable venders and tourists, and carrying their weapons in innocent-looking packages. Within a day of the Offensive, the VC had penetrated the American Embassy, rocking the stability of American power, and sending shock waves into the White House in Washington and to every American home via television. The battle raged for nearly a month, with the main fighting during the first ten days. The Communists had appalling losses–estimated between 50,000 – 70,000 killed and wounded, whilst the Allies suffered some 10,000 casualties.

* * *

Digging my shell-scrape was now a major ordeal for me. With no energy through lack of eating because of the severe nausea, even the simplest tasks seemed overwhelming. Sitting against a tree, staring into nothingness, I felt totally discouraged and depressed. Every time I was forced to relieve myself, because of the diarrhoea, I felt my spirit draining away and my physical strength with the black fluid that poured out of my body. The only positive thought was that 'thank God for the Tet holiday and for a few days' rest from the fighting.

The next morning, I woke feeling a little better, and ate a small breakfast. The previous day's rest had restored me a little. At mid-morning, there was a strange feeling in the air and a low rumbling of artillery fire away in the distance could be heard. All the section commanders called their men together for an urgent briefing. We sat on the ground, surrounding Paul as he spoke.

"The Tet holiday has been cancelled," he informed us. "Charlie's gone berserk and is trying to take over the whole f_ckin' country. They've taken out the Yank Embassy in Saigon. So, pack up, we're moving out in an hour's time. We're heading north of here to secure a new chopper pad for resupply. Fill in your shell-scrapes and get ready on the double."

The following day, having secured a landing zone, we were resupplied with rations and extra ammunition for the expected coming battle and precious water. At midday, we crossed a river and headed northwest towards where B Company was positioned.

In the middle of the afternoon, sounds of heavy fighting were heard coming from B Company's position, 2000 metres away. Apparently, they had found an enemy camp and attacked it, but had been repulsed with heavy casualties. V Company was ordered to move quickly to support them and then take over the attack early the next morning. We travelled through thick jungle, in record time, putting our lead scouts in greater danger with the increased pace.

We reached their location just before dusk, tired, but ready to fight. The rest two days earlier had lifted my spirits and my strength and could keep up in the forced march. I felt excited by the thought of the coming battle, probably because of the contrast of how terrible I felt two days earlier.

On arrival, we took over B Company's positions, as they organised themselves to withdraw. I climbed into a freshly dug trench occupied by two young, white-faced Australians.

"You okay, Digger?" I asked.

"Hell, are we bloody glad to see you blokes," one replied in a shaky voice. For the next 30 minutes, we conversed in whispers as brothers in arms that were comforting and uplifting for the three of us.

After B Company had recovered their dead, and wounded, they withdrew and formed a harbour 200 metres away. Soon after, we fell back into the harbour that they had formed. It was dark when we pulled back and found it difficult moving through the thick jungle to link up with our Australian brothers. Challenging as it was, we finally managed. Even though it was cramped with so many men in the confined space, it was very comforting. Particularly for the Aussies, having been in a serious fight that afternoon. Forming defensive harbours at night was not only necessary for protection but also good for morale.

Throughout the night, heavy NVA mortar fire landed on our former position, and it was comforting to know that our commanders knew what they were doing in pulling us back. We could only wonder at how many casualties we would have suffered had we remained there, judging from the concentrated bombardment that came in 200 metres away.

That night, most of us did not sleep well, for we knew that the next morning might be our last as each man contemplated the coming attack on the enemy camp. I lay in my shell-scrape, listening to the silence between the mortar attacks and the disturbing sounds of men in troubled sleep all around me. It was strange how quiet the jungle was after the sounds of battle had stopped.

'Tomorrow I may die.' I thought, unemotionally. I wondered if this was how my uncles felt before they went into battle against the Germans in the Second World War? Particularly, my Uncle Max, who fought in the jungles of New Guinea against the Japanese. 'What will tomorrow bring? Will I still be alive this time tomorrow night to have such thoughts?'

Early next morning, while it was still dark, the stillness allowed a light mist to cling to the tops of the surrounding trees. In the semi-darkness, I could barely see the man standing in front, as we all stood in single file on the track, waiting for the order to move towards our attack positions. Each man stood alone, fully prepared for battle, with rifle at the ready. Some had fixed bayonets, and most had hand grenades hanging from webbing for quick use. No one spoke, and final last-minute instructions were passed down the line to each man in quiet whispers, acknowledged with a nod, and then quietly passed on.

I was glad that Stuart had been sent to Company HQ and would be out of harm's way.

I turned and looked at the guy standing behind me. He was nervously moving one foot back and forth, then looked up, sensing my gaze. I sent him a weak, encouraging smile, which I wasn't sure he saw in the dim light. He nodded to assure me he was okay. I nodded back and turned, facing grimly up the track, where we would soon all be moving.

It was February 1st, and I was twenty-two years old that day. 'Will I die on my birthday?' I wondered, yet I was not consciously afraid. The old SAS trick before a mission was to accept that I will die and that all I need is to focus on doing my job and take as many of the enemy with me. In hindsight, this may be an effective strategy to perform an impossible task and perhaps avoid emotional trauma. But I suspect it was just another way of suppressing real feelings, which would create huge psychological damage. Years later, this very event played out in one of my healing sessions, suggesting that I had emotionally hurt myself.

Besides, a greater concern for me was the state of my deteriorating health. My head felt as if it were splitting in two. My stomach was in painful knots from diarrhoea cramps and no doubt from anxiety of the coming attack. Already since waking, I had relieved myself three times.

Because of the strict water rationing because of the military situation, and resupply being uncertain, cleaning teeth or even washing face or hands was forbidden since the cancellation of the Tet holiday. I looked down at my hands. They were filthy from dust, sweat, and human waste. I dared not touch my unshaven face for fear of passing on germs that festered on the grime of sticky, blackened fingers. Each time my guts gave me the undeniable message to empty my bowels, I would quickly take ten steps to find some privacy, drop my pants and let the black liquid run out of my body. As terrible as I felt, I was determined to excrete in private and preserve what little dignity remained. It would have been so easy to have given up and let it all go in my pants. Each time I dropped them; the odour that assailed my nostrils nearly caused me to throw up. I'd long given up wearing underpants, thus allowing air to circulate around my vital parts, which slightly reduced the stench.

"Okay, you blokes, this is it," came the whispered command. "It's just us. The Aussies are staying here, and we're taking the camp on our own. So, move out, Six Platoon leading."

We quietly moved up the hill towards the unknown of what may lie in wait for us at the top of the hill. The early morning briefing raced through my mind, already going crazy from a mixture of physical pain, emotional excitement, and fear. The plan was for Six Platoon to lead the attack and take the left portion of the enemy camp at the top of the crest. Then we were to form a fire base, allowing Four and Five Platoons to take out the rest of the camp in a flanking attack. This plan, though, could go seriously wrong if the VC had been reinforced during the night.

Half-way up the hill, the crest dissolved in fire and steel as several US aircraft flew close over us and dropped their high explosive bombs, napalm fireball bombs and rockets on to the enemy position. This coincided with massive artillery fire from our guns back in fire-base Anderson, landing on the same target. We all sat where we were fully alert and waited. The artillery barrage lasted for over ten minutes. This gave me the opportunity to attend to the demand to empty my bowels yet again. As the barrage stopped, we started moving towards the top of the crest.

Just short of the top of the hill, we spread out to prepare for the assault. A deathly silence followed the terrible destruction that had rained down upon the enemy positions. I passed one of our blokes, who looked at me in quiet anxiety.

"This is a 'ropey one,' Sas." (Not a good situation). His whispered voice was hoarse and choking. I nodded grimly and walked on.

In an extended line, we began slowly and silently moving, crouched over through the thick undergrowth towards the enemy positions.

Suddenly, the top of the hill, thirty metres above us, erupted in massive explosions as two more US jets swooped in and dropped their bombs. We all dived for cover as shrapnel whirled about, snapping branches and leaves off trees that fell on us. A napalm fireball bomb that engulfed an enemy position so close directly above us mostly shook me. This would be part of a nightmare I would have every night for many years to come.

We hadn't heard them coming, as they were travelling so fast until they had passed over us. The timing of their attack was obviously uncoordinated by the airstrike and artillery bombardment minutes earlier. No one was hurt and several guys were shaking their heads that summed up the danger from so-called supporting fire and how lucky we were yet again (the third time) had been inaccurately timed or placed.

Hamish Wilson gave the silent signal, and we quietly crept forward, then stopped one last time to prepare for the attack. We lay down in a firing position in readiness for whatever may happen next. Then the order came!

"Charge," We leapt to our feet. Over the lip of the hill, we charged with fixed bayonets, covering the last few metres that separated us from the enemy camp. Bunkers greeted us, but mercifully, not the expected gunfire. The artillery fire and air strikes had destroyed many bunkers and trenches. Several were fiercely burning from the napalm.

On reaching each bunker, we tossed in grenades and ran in immediately after the explosion, ready to kill anything that was still alive. All fear had vanished, being caught up in the excitement of the moment. Every bunker was empty. It seemed that the VC had pulled out minutes before the attack.

We formed our fire base, as Four, and Five Platoons attacked from their positions. They ran into some retreating enemy from our part of the camp and fought their way into the far side of the enemy base. Within minutes, the remaining Communists realised their hopeless position and fled, taking their dead and wounded with them.

As the last shots died away, it became uncannily quiet. A pall of smoke from grenades, gunfire and a small grassfire settled over the camp. The rank smell of cordite hung in the air.

Suddenly, a lone VC ran out from one of the bunkers we had already searched and began to raise his arms, perhaps intending to surrender. His sudden appearance caused highly strung nerves to react, and he was instantly gunned down, dying immediately. Within seconds, another VC began firing from a bunker that also had been searched. Several members of Four Platoon crawled up to the bunker and threw in grenades. The VC crawled out screaming, with one leg blown completely off. He was quickly bayoneted to death. The battle was finally over, and miraculously, we had suffered no casualties, except for shattered nerves.

The camp was now thoroughly searched. We found a complete field hospital with blood transfusion kits, operating equipment and a mountain of drugs and food. A number of weapons and a lot of ammunition were also captured.

All the drugs, transfusion kits and equipment were stacked and later blown up. The weapons and ammunition were carried away and flown out by helicopter. The food was given out to those that wanted it. Amongst the food were several cartons of French condensed milk. As a boy, I had read about Charles Upham, the New Zealand double Victoria Cross winner in the Second World War, and how he had coped with dysentery by living off just condensed milk. This had enabled him to keep going through the thick of the fighting. Recalling this, I grabbed four cans and consumed them all throughout the day. I could eat nothing else, and it was good to get something back into my stomach. By midday, however, I was relieving myself every ten minutes and was becoming dreadfully dehydrated from so much liquid loss from my body.

We moved off the hill to a position about 800 metres away and formed a harbour. Walking to this new position was almost beyond my strength, and I was forced to stop and rest every few metres. Several friends offered to carry my pack, but I refused. My pride demanded that I see this through. I'd lost a terrible amount of weight and my reserves were nearly exhausted. 'If I survive this hell, I'm going to find myself the safest job in the world when I get home,' was my strongest thought.

After arriving at the new location and settled in, about 1750 hours, 4 VC were sighted by sentries of 5 platoon, 30 metres away. They were allowed to approach to about 15 metres before being fired upon. The first VC was killed, the second was wounded and returned fire, while the rest disappeared back down the track. Except for Des Hirini, the sentries withdrew under cover from the M60 machine gun that suddenly jammed. The wounded VC continued with his AK47 automatic fire. Des, who was sheltering behind a tree, moved out from his shelter to fire back. But being left-handed exposed the full right side of his body. The VC quickly saw him and fired and Des was killed instantly.

Several guys rushed out to Des's position, found him dead, and reported back. Every man in Five Platoon stood up, feeling shocked and angry. Sensing the mood of his men, their Platoon Commander, Graye Shattky, made a snap decision. To his section commanders gathered around him he uttered only three words:

"Go get 'em."

In seething rage, the three sections of 5 Platoon fanned out at the run in three different directions, with only one intent – to avenge their fallen mate.

The wounded VC became trapped between two converging sections and died in a hail of bullets from twenty incensed men. They continued firing at the fallen figure until their anger and magazines were exhausted and left an unrecognizable, bloodied heap. The third section ran into another VC and badly wounded him, but he escaped, leaving a trail of blood. Two weapons were captured. Des was carried back in a body bag. We all felt sad to lose him, for he was popular throughout the entire company.

By nightfall, all was quiet again. I was feeling very ill both from the taste of the condensed milk in my mouth and from its effect on my stomach. Because of the poor state of my health, I was relieved from sentry duty, but I couldn't sleep. Around midnight it seemed as if my body was falling apart and I vomited for nearly an hour, mostly dry retching, as there was nothing left in me to bring up.

Next morning, whilst dozing in my shell scrape, I opened my eyes to see the outline of Hamish Wilson standing over me. The sun was behind him, dazzling my eyes. I sat up, and he crouched beside me.

"How are you feeling, Sisson?"

"Not good, sir."

"Do you think you can carry on?" I looked at him, in a blank and uncomprehending way. Intuitively, I knew that my life was held delicately in the balance and would be decided in the next few seconds of conversation. My pride exerted itself. It felt that if I were to leave this hellhole, I would be failing, and to stay would mean an uncertain future. My options were simple and yet I felt very confused. Slowly, I shook my head, resigning myself to whatever fate had in store for me. "I don't know. I don't know anything anymore, sir."

"Umm. I think perhaps you should be taken out on the next chopper. There's one coming in later this morning to take Des and the captured weapons to Firebase Anderson. I want you on it, okay?"

"Yes sir," I heard myself say with a sigh of resignation.

As Wilson walked away, I buried my face in my jungle hat as if to hide it, unsure if I was feeling shame or relief.

12
DUST OFF

It was late morning, and the 'dust off' helicopter hovered thirty metres above the ground, just above the treetops. Des's body and the captured weapons were winched up first.

The lone VC sniper* moved carefully towards the sound of the hovering helicopter, knowing he could get a good shot without being detected because of the engine noise. Slowly moving closer, not to be seen by enemy troops, he finally got a clear view of a body being winched up, then it got caught up in the branches, freed, only to get caught again. It was taking long, increasing his opportunity, but he could not see the helicopter above the trees. He knew he could have a clear shot if a live person was winched up or down and if no target presented itself, he could always try to take the chopper out by firing at the sound of its engines.

I stood waiting for Des's body to be disconnected from the winch aboard the Huey and then lowered again through the branches for me. This operation was taking longer than any of us wanted as the threat of snipers was always a danger. Blue was standing beside me to help, and as the saddle of the winch appeared through the trees, he quickly and thoroughly wrapped it around my body securely. With no clear view of the Huey directly above us, our radio operator informed the aircrew to hoist me up.

"Get yourself well, mate." Blue yelled above the engine noise as I lifted towards the hovering Huey.

"You stay safe, Blue." I yelled back.

I too was getting caught in the branches on the way up but could untangle myself allowing the winch to keep pulling me upwards. Twice I

---

* An estimate of probably what happened.

got seriously caught and on freeing myself made me and the winch swing wildly from side to side.

Suddenly there was a loud cracking sound, not unlike a bullet travelling close above my head. I peered upwards and concluded that the Huey's engine was back-firing. Then a second 'crack' followed with a third seconds later. I frantically looked up to see what was happening. The winch pulled me up more quickly. Seconds later, I was nearing the tops of the trees. The Huey seemed to backfire several more times and rocked violently. It suddenly revved its engines, banked to the left and raced away, dragging me dangling five metres below through the treetops. Fortunately, at that height there were no large branches and 5 seconds later I reached the open door and two pairs of hands pulled me inside.

"Are you okay?" the Australian aircrewman shouted into my ear over the noise of the engines as he unbuckled the harness. "I think so. What the hell was that all about?" I shouted back. He smiled at me and motioned for me to sit on the floor.

Twenty minutes later, we landed at Fire Base Anderson. I climbed out of the Huey, thanking the air crew for getting me safely here. I hobbled to the side of the landing zone, dazed and disorientated. After finding the nearest latrine, I returned and sat down beside the airfield, vacantly watching the local activity of men hurrying past and helicopters constantly coming and going.

Half an hour later, I recognized the familiar face of Brian O'Conner, one of our Company HQ NCOs, as he walked over to me.

"We heard you got wounded being lifted out."

"Apart from a bloody guts ache, I'm okay. Why?"

"Did you know your chopper was hit three times by a sniper'?"

"What? Are you kidding me?"

"You didn't know that a sniper was trying to get you?"

"Bloody hell no!" I answered.

"Yeah. The pilot told me that the bastard was trying to hit you but couldn't because you were swaying too much. So, he tried to knock the bloody chopper out of the sky. The aircrew thought you knew and were swaying the harness on purpose. We thought you'd been hit, judging by all the excitement from the chopper crew."

I looked at the ground and shook my head.

"Bugger me," was all I could mutter. I realized that the cracking sounds were the sound of the sniper's bullets passing close overhead. I should have known, as I had heard that cracking sound enough times already.

"Anyway, I'm here to take you to 'RAP' (Regimental Aid Post) for a medical. Let's go. The jeep's over here."

An hour later, I found myself stripped off and being examined by an Australian doctor. He was unusually talkative, and I was happy with that, as I found talking exhausting.

"You're a sick boy. How long have you had these symptoms?"

"For nearly a week," I answered.

"Well, my lad, you certainly don't have diarrhoea. It looks like you have full-blow amoebic dysentery. That's why your shit is black, because it's blood. There's no way of checking it here, but they can do that in Nui Dat. You should be in hospital, but there's not a hospital bed left in the country. Those that are still available are being reserved for the seriously wounded. We've had so many casualties in the last few days, we don't know where to put them all. Two days ago, we had a young guy brought in unconscious, shot through the throat, and his 'dog tags' were missing, probably shot off. We didn't know if he was a Yank or one of our own blokes, so we shipped him to Saigon. Last I heard, he was on a plane to Hawaii. I guess they will sort it out when this bloody lot's over." He paused for a moment, as if reflecting on the nightmare we were all in. Then continued.

"Okay, as for you, you can go back to Nui Dat by the next available chopper. The medics there will take care of you. You'll have to sleep in your own tent. Take these tablets as prescribed on the label and it will stop the runs. It won't cure you, but you'll start feeling a lot better in a few days. They'll probably ship you back home, or to Malaysia, where I think your base is. Make sure you report there to your regimental doctor. You need proper treatment in a hospital. This will only keep you going until you are out of Vietnam, so be glad you are out of the war in reasonably one piece. By the way, try to get back to Nut Dat before tonight. Intelligence thinks Charlie's going to try to take this base out in an attack, and probably tonight. There's a huge NVA unit, probably a battalion, maybe even a regiment strength heading this way, and there are no allied reserves left to stop them. Good luck. Who's next?"

Brain took me back to his tent where he gave me some fresh bread, water, and I downed two of the tablets, while we exchanged news.

"We've got a big fight on our hands with this lot," he informed me.

"There's heavy fighting all over the country. Shit, it's really big. Parts of Saigon have been taken and much of Hue." He continued. "But Charlie is taking a real hammering in all areas. I'm sure we'll hold them, but they're bloody determined.

Anyway, enough talk. You'll want a shower. It must have been ten days since you had one. They are not much, but the Engineers set them up with 44-gallon drums with holes in the bottom and they are good and hot. I'll show you where they are."

"Oh, yes please, but what's this about Charlie possibly hitting Anderson 'tonight?"

"We don't know for sure, but an enemy unit large enough to easily over-run us is not far away, and every available friendly unit is fully tied down just holding their own ground. So, we just might see something tonight. Are you going to still be here?"

"I hope bloody not."

I had the showers to myself and noticed with delight that there was hot water ready to go. I stripped off and threw away my now rotting clothes. Brain had secured a replacement new uniform from stores.

My skin was dirty white and wrinkly, as if it had been submerged in water for a long period. I noticed my hands were shaking. My bones stuck out, with little flesh left to cover them. What an incredible delight to have hot water run over my wasted body made me nearly cry with joy.

An hour later, I was back waiting beside the landing zone for the next available flight to Nui Dat. Choppers were coming and going all afternoon, but there was never an available space for me. I felt a growing fear, as I was desperate to get out before nightfall. My sanity couldn't handle any further combat was something I was sure about.

All the defences around Anderson were being reinforced to prepare for the expected attack. I could see the 105mm artillery guns being repositioned and lowering their muzzles horizontally from their normal upright position. When one of the Aussie gunners who was passing stopped when I enquired what they were doing. He explained it was to prepare for the use of shrapnel shells.

"Each gun will become a huge claymore mine that we can keep loading and blasting the hell out of Charlie."

"Wow, that will stop them dead in their tracks." I uttered.

"The first wave or two, but if the force is as big as they think, it will only slow them down." He gloomily replied.

I might have been ready to die for my country at the beginning of the operation. Right now, survival was the most important thing, and staying in Firebase Anderson would not enhance that option. 'I have to get out,' was my strongest thought.

As each hour passed, my increasing anxiety made itself physically known; I spent most of my time going back and forth to the latrine.

Father Burke, a Catholic priest whom I'd met in Nui Dat a month earlier, found me by the airfield and sat down to talk.

"You don't look too good," he commented. Our conversation was very comforting. It was good to share my fears about not getting out by nightfall. While we talked, a captured NVA major was carried past on a stretcher. He'd been shot in both legs and was being sent back to Nui Dat for interrogation and an uncertain future.

Before leaving to continue his duties, he tried to re-assure me.

"I'm sure you will be out by tonight. You'll be ok."

Soon after, a kind-faced older Australian sergeant sat down beside me to talk. After my chats with these two men, I felt my spirits lift considerably, along with fewer trips to the latrine, signalling that the tablets were working.

By 6.30pm in the growing darkness, the last chopper out of Firebase Anderson was about to leave. I hobbled over to it.

"Can you please squeeze me in?" I pleaded.

"Sorry mate. We are completely full," the pilot yelled back.

I looked at the pilot, my hopes fading, as it stood ready to lift off, filled with personal not needed for the coming battle. Close to despair, knowing that when this chopper left, I would be stuck here until the next day – except that there might not be a next day for Anderson.

I turned away and walked back to the edge of the airfield, feeling totally numb to await my fate. Dropping my pack and webbing, sat down and considered my options over the next 10 to 12 hours. I watched the helicopter that was now lifting off on its way to Nui Dat. 'There goes my only hope. Perhaps I should have stayed with the company and taken my chances with them, after all.'

Suddenly, the helicopter stopped ascending and re-landed. In the semidarkness, I saw the familiar figure of Father Burke jump off the Huey and run towards me.

"Here, son, you take my place on the chopper. You probably have a mother that loves you and I don't want her grieving tomorrow."

He bent down and helped me to my feet, and carrying my pack and holding one arm, led me to the chopper. He yelled into my ear, above the noise of the engines, as I climbed on board. "Besides, if there's an attack tonight, I wouldn't mind a bit of a punch-up." Looking more seriously, directly into my eyes.

"Survive this war. Good luck, son."

The Huey took off as soon as I was aboard. I was so overcome with emotion to utter a single word, and managed only a simple wave, which he may not have seen. 'You may be giving your life for me,' was my only thought. Never had I felt such relief and gratitude.

The chopper levelled out at 2000 metres, safe from enemy ground fire. It was turning dark. In every direction, as far as the eye could see, the ground was lit up like a gigantic firework display as battles raged. It was particularly intense, about fifteen kilometres away to the east of Anderson, where a massive battle was in progress. The unmistakable blue-green tracer bullets of the Communist and our own reddish/orange-coloured tracers could be clearly seen tearing into each other. Flashes of light pinpointed the explosions of grenades, shells, and mortar rounds. Men were dying down there amid the dust, sweat, blood and fear. It was the closest glimpse into hell I had ever seen.

An hour later, we touched down at Nui Dat. Colin Burgering met me from our platoon. He had remained at Nui Dat as with each operation a small number were selected to be rested and help defend Nui Dat.

"Welcome back, Sas. The jeep's over here. We heard you'd been wounded.

"Nope, just one big guts ache," I replied.

"Keep your rifle handy tonight. A captured Charlie has escaped and is running loose somewhere in the camp."

That was one thing I didn't want to hear! Colin dropped me off in our deserted and darkened line of tents. I fumbled my way into my own, carefully checking it for any unwelcome intruders – man or beast. I found my way in the dark to the latrines and then had a quick shower, gripping my rifle all the time. Back in my tent, I tied a piece of string across the entrance at knee height to act as a tripwire. I then connected the string to the trigger of my rifle, in which I tied to my stretcher, aimed at chest height, directly at the only entrance into the tent. If anyone tries to come in, they will be blown away. I slipped the safety-catch off.

Years later, I realised that taking this precaution had been foolish, as it would have endangered any friend or medic who might have wanted to check up on me during the night. Such an accidental death would have been tragic and me being court marshalled on a charge of manslaughter. But then, I was so fearful and felt I was fighting for my very life against a hostile world. With one hand on my rifle and the other gripping my unsheathed bayonet gave me a sense of comfort.

The thought trickled into my mind, 'what if I cut myself on my bayonet during sleep? It is very sharp. There are worse things that could happen to me this night.' I felt an anger well up in me and contemplated what I would do to the VC with my bayonet if he came into my tent and survived my booby trap. The thoughts were too grotesque and ugly to print here. But within a minute, something got released, and I suddenly felt empowered. The words of my instructor back on the interrogation and torture training with the SAS filtered into my mind.

"No matter how bad your situation is, if you feel in control, you will feel empowered, and no situation or person will break you."

I felt in control of my life for the first time in weeks, if not months. It felt strange and uplifting. I drifted into sleep wondering if I would have my usual nightmares of burning to death by napalm and seeing myself lying dead with a bullet hole in my face.

I opened my eyes, with the sun streaming through the ventilation strip in the tent, well past the usual company 'Stand to' at first light. I had been woken by the arrival of one of the company medics.

"Hold it, don't come in," I yelled, sliding quickly from my stretcher, slipping on the safety-catch of my rifle, and cutting the 'trip-wire' string with my bayonet. He didn't notice his danger, nor my foolishness. Doing so I noticed that even though I'd had lots of dreams, but no nightmares and I felt refreshed, despite the nausea feeling in my stomach. Unfortunately, the nightmares were to return the next night and would continue for many years.

I was happy to hear later in the day that Fire-Base Anderson wasn't attacked the previous night as expected, but was heavily shelled and suffered a number of casualties. I was later to happily discover that Father Burke was not one of them. However, a village one kilometre down the road, held by a battalion of ARVN, became the target instead and was completely routed and overrun. It totally wiped one ARVN infantry company of nearly 200 men out, another surrendered, changing sides, and joining the Communists. The rest of the battalion escaped and most deserted. Two days later, the village was retaken by the Americans after air strikes had levelled it.

The next five days were spent in having a series of medical tests, medication, a lot of sleeping, fewer visits to the latrine and eventually eating again. As each day passed, I felt my strength returning, thanks to modern drugs. The doctor echoed the words of his colleague at Anderson, reminding me to report to the hospital on my return to Malaysia, which will be on the next available flight. I was so happy to be leaving Vietnam.

At one of the doctor's visits, I mentioned my experience of everything slowing down and feeling incredibly joyful in the middle of a battle. I had been too ashamed to mention it to any of my friends or to a doctor before this, having concluded that it was a sign of insanity. The doctor replied.

"So, the feeling of deep euphoria and probably the slowing down of everything was just a sign of intense stress. That's all and it will soon pass after you go home. Nothing to worry about."

I felt he didn't really understand what I was saying but was happy at his explanation.

"So, I'm not going crazy?" He hesitated too long before answering.

"Um, ah, no. It is normal for this to happen to you guys going through so much combat. You will be okay."

He was unconvincing, and I became even more certain that this was a sign that I was losing my sanity and never mentioned it again to anyone out of shame. To be sent home as unfit for combat duty would be, for me, the ultimate disgrace.

The next day I was shocked to learn that my shipping out orders had been cancelled. The decision was made because there were some signs of my recovery and because of the high number of casualties to V Company. Instead, I would be returned to active duty as soon as possible. By February 10, although still very weak, I was medically passed as fit enough for combat duty. I suspect I was passed only because of the military situation. I found out later that anyone with the serious condition of dysentery that I had is hospitalized. I returned by helicopter to re-join V company.

13
THE BATTLE

During my convalescence, V Company had been involved in a lot of combat. Every day they had engagements with VC and NVA units, the most notable occurring on February 7, with a major battle. After speaking with those willing to talk about it, including Barry Toohill, along with Tony Howell's outstanding book, 'Jungle Green Shadows,' I could piece together what happened.

The battle was with a large enemy force and its size was under contention, ranging from a full battalion, 400–600 Communist soldiers down to 50 men (small company size) which Major Worsnop stated in his battle report. Brian Worsnop was renowned for his modest reporting, preferring to understate his achievements. My reason for doubting this smaller number is found in Communist battle tactics, which state that an attacking force must always have a 3 to 1 ratio advantage or more over the enemy. Most armies throughout the world also have this as a basic offensive policy. The VC would have been well informed of the strength of V Company, being approximately 130 men. Also in Tony Howell's book, put the figure at being a battalion size. Intelligence reports after the battle from documents found on the bodies revealed they were members of Viet Cong mainline 3 Battalion of 274 Regiment, comprising 3 rifle companies, one support company and large elements of NVA (North Vietnamese Army) troops. The following account from members of V Company strongly suggests that this was more accurate.

Communist preparation for battle

V company had formed a triangular all-round defence near the location of a contact the day before, where one New Zealander was killed.

In the dark early hours of the 7th, the Communists moved in, intending to wipe out the smaller force of a prized ANZAC Company. As the enemy crept in to set up fire bases surrounding the New Zealanders prior to their main attack, they could not move silently. The thick jungle terrain was difficult enough to noiselessly move through during the day, and in the quiet darkness amplified the sound of all movement. They were so loud, particularly in front of 4 and 6 platoon, that many members of V Company assumed a herd of domestic water buffalo, bullocks or wild pigs caused the noise seeking water that was nearby.

Six platoon went on 50% 'stand to' in readiness just in case. The noise directly in front of 4 Platoon caused Tony Howell, 4 platoon commander, to become convinced that it was a huge enemy force moving into position to prepare for a major attack. He called his platoon to 'stand to' in readiness and informed Company HQ of his concerns. By this time, the enemy movement was so close to 4 Platoon's position and from the sound of such a large force that if they launched an attack, V Company could easily be overrun and wiped out. A Communist victory on this scale would have tremendous psychological effect and would be the biggest New Zealand military disaster since World War Two.

In total darkness, the time being 0615, Tony Howell decided to fire the claymores along his front opposite the VC, moving into position. With a deafening explosion, the claymore mines wreaked their destruction of thousands of lethal ball bearings, blasting their way through the jungle foliage, destroying everything in their path. This action probably saved the company from annihilation.

Four Platoon

Thinking that the element of surprise had been lost, which it already had 15 minutes earlier, the VC Commander ordered the attack to begin, earlier than planned, which would have been at first light. With the sound of a burgle signalling to attack the VC company opposite, 4 platoon sprang into action with their weapons blasting, charged through the undergrowth with only one intention. They were heavily supported by a strong firebase on their flank, with fire from machine guns and RPGs (rocket propelled grenades). The claymore mines had decimated the first wave before they had even started. Then the second and third wave instantly became pinned down before they had coved 5–10 metres by the M60 machine guns, rifle and M79 grenade launcher fire of 4 platoon. The intensity and closeness of the contact was overwhelming, with both sides determined to hold the line.

The initial danger of being overrun was blunted, and both sides exchanged a relentless withering fire to win the firefight.

The artillery

Once the battle began, artillery defensive fire was called in front of 4 platoon. But it was not until about 6.25 am, before the artillery had air clearance and could open fire (ensuring there were no aircraft or helicopters flying in the area that could be hit). It was about 10 full minutes that 4 platoon fought a desperate fight unsupported.

19-year-old Barry Toohill, the artillery forward observer, kept a cool head and did a battle saving job of bringing the artillery rounds from the Australian 108 Field battery onto the location directly in front of 4 Platoon. Normally an officer's role, Toohill was given the task several days earlier, being the only one available. By radio, Toohill talked to 108 Field Artillery, guiding the incoming exploding shells and crept the fire ever closer to 4 platoon intending to engulf the VC front units. Tony Howell was asked via radio from 108 Field battery if the fire was close enough. He called out to his men if they wanted the artillery fire to come in closer. He got a resounding "Yes," which highlighted the desperation of the situation for the New Zealanders.

By now, the shells were exploding as close as 25 metres from 4 platoon and some even closer. The front VC units were now coming under direct artillery fire. Some leapt to their feet and charged, only to be cut down by returning gunfire, if not by the exploding shells.

Heavy fire from the VC supporting firebase continued, much of the RPGs firing high and bursting in the trees, showering 4 platoon with shrapnel and sharp wooden splinters. Some of the VC fire was overshooting 4 Platoon and landing behind on to V Company HQ, positioned in the middle of the all-round defence. By now, fire from the VC in front of 4 platoon was lessening as their losses mounted and it was becoming clear that for now, they were unable to push home their attack. This was probably the time when the VC started clearing their dead and wounded while maintaining suppressive cover fire.

It was revealed after the battle that most of the VC had a cloth cord around their necks, enabling them to be easily dragged from the area when seriously wounded or killed to hide from the allies their actual casualty numbers. We had seen this before when encountering larger VC units, but here, almost every one of them had a drag cord around their necks. This showed that the VC and NVA expected a victory with heavy losses.

Five Platoon

With the attack in front of 4 platoon stalled, the VC launched phase two of the battle. At approximately 0635 hours, with burgles sounding again signalled the attack against 5 platoon as waves of VC opened fire with automatic gunfire, charged. They too were heavily supported by RPG's and machine gun fire from their already established firebase on their flank.

It was still dark with a little light creeping in, but sight was still limited because of the smoke and both sides had to rely on firing at their enemy muzzle flashes from their weapons.

The assault on 5 Platoon was just as ferocious as against 4 Platoon, as the VC probed for any weaknesses in the perimeter as they tried to locate and overrun the forward defences. The firing of 5 platoon's claymores decimated the first VC wave, but quickly replaced by a second and third wave. Good fire discipline, desperate determination with the artillery help enabled V Company to hold on.

Barry Toohill now redirected 108 Field fire from 4 platoon to 5 platoon's front. With a brief pause with this shift of artillery support, the VC were able to get alarmingly close to 5 Platoons defences before being pinned down by the relentless fire.

Having cleared their casualties, and replaced their losses with backup teams, the enemy renewed their attack on 4 platoon, and now the battle was raging on two fronts. The situation was approaching a climax for both sides. V Company was disturbingly close to being overrun because of the closeness of the VC front line, as close as 5 metres in some places. Yet only the determination and unrelenting fire from the New Zealanders held the line. Both sides were on a knife edge and the battle could go either way.

The VC displayed many of the classical jungle warfare tactics V Company had trained in back in Malaysia: 'fire and movement,' trying to eliminate the M60 machine guns by throwing hand grenades and directed RPG fire on to them just to name a couple. This was no ordinary irregular unit we normally came up against. These were well trained, battle-hardened veteran regulars.

The incoming artillery in front of 5 platoon had similar results as with 4 platoon's front. One difficulty now was that the trajectory height and location of 5 platoon made the 'creeping of fire' towards their front much more difficult and some shells were hitting the tops of the trees as they passed overhead, showering shrapnel down on the men below causing casualties on friend or foe alike.

Toohill was now offered additional help from 2 RAR 81mm mortars stationed in Firebase Anderson, Southeast of V Company's position. Also, another battery of 105mm guns became available as well as fire from a battery of the huge American 175mm guns. With shell explosions far greater than 108's guns, Toohill kept the 175mm fire at a safer distance to harass the enemy rear.

With the artillery fire creeping ever so close to the forward VC units, each Communist commander knew that to stay pinned down in their present position would mean that eventually they would be engulfed and annihilated. Other alternatives would be to withdraw back through the artillery fire, costing more casualties or press home their attacks. Many chose the latter, resulting in appalling losses for these VC front units. VC tactics would ensure that these front decimated units would have backup troops waiting behind to replace them.

Throughout this, the company and platoon medics were crawling among and administering to the mounting number of New Zealand wounded. Lou Phillips and Ron Prichard repeatedly went to many of the wounded and treated them while under fire. Ron was awarded the Distinguished Conduct Medal (DCM) for his bravery. He and Lou should have both received the Victoria Cross, the British Commonwealth and New Zealand's highest award for bravery in the face of the enemy.

The battle had been raging for 35 minutes, and ammunition was dwindling. It was getting lighter, and V Company could now see more clearly, inflicting even more casualties on the enemy and making every bullet count. The VC could also now see more clearly, and the casualties on both sides continued to mount.

Six Platoon

At approximately 0650 hours, phase three of the enemy battle plan was launched. With burgles sounding again, the VC company opposite 6 platoon sprang into the attack. The initial assault was temporarily halted with the firing of 6 platoon's claymores with devastating results. Then gathered pace as a second and third wave joined in the charge.

Now V company was being attacked from all sides. The stakes had gone up an extra notch. Many inexperienced defenders and some ARVN units against such a determined Communist thrust would have panicked, run, or surrendered at this point. This is what the VC were no doubt waiting for. Even if one or two New Zealanders panicked and ran could spell disaster for the entire company.

Being surrounded, with at least the three to one ratio disadvantage, with no means of retreat, was not a good military situation to be in for a defensive unit. There are only three choices: win, surrender or be overrun. Being overrun generally means that all defenders are killed. There can be no stalemate or draw in this situation. Also, none of the defenders had any idea or concerned themselves about the size of the enemy force and stayed focused on doing their job. There simply was no time for anyone to consider the appalling danger they were in. One can only wonder what was running through Major Workshop's mind. No doubt he had complete faith in his men.

Because of the thick impenetrable bamboo covering half of 6 Platoon's front, the enemy attack was more concentrated and therefore more intense on only two sections of the Platoon. But this also acted as a bottleneck against the VC, allowing the New Zealanders a more concentrated return fire with two M60 machine guns, along with half of the Platoon's rifleman and M79 grenade launchers. Hamish Wilson (platoon commander) ordered the repositioning of a third M60 to be added to the fight. This quickly stalled the attack, causing the VC to become pinned down like their comrades on the other two sides of the battle.

Eddie Tataurangi, the mortar forward observer, took over directing the mortar fire from Toohill and brought the fire onto 6 platoon's front and crept the exploding rounds into as close as 20 metres from the perimeter with devastating effect on the VC.

The Australian B Company, our old friend from the battle a week earlier, was ordered to travel and link up with V Company to relieve the pressure. Being too far away could not arrive in time.

There were so many acts of heroism on both sides that to include them would take an entire book on this engagement alone.

By about 0730 hours, it was light enough to bring in helicopter gunships to take over from the artillery and mortar fire, lessening the danger to our own troops of exploding shells in treetops and blasting shrapnel. Two heavily armed AH-1 Cobra helicopter gunships with forward firing 7.62 mini-guns and 70 mm Zuni rockets strafed and pounded the remaining enemy still engaged in the firefight that raged on every front surrounding V Company. Their heavy firepower was even more accurate and effective and could be brought in even closer than the artillery.

This finally broke the back of the Communist attack. With nowhere to hide from the circling gunships and the intensity of their firepower, combined with V Company's relentless fire, the VC and NVA hastily evacuated all their wounded and most of their dead, then disengaged and retreated. By about 0815, the battle was over.

Only thirteen VC bodies were found, but from the many drag marks and blood-trails, it was obvious that the enemy had taken a terrible beating. V Company suffered only ten wounded in the battle, three seriously and miraculously, no fatalities. A large amount of ammunition, weapons and equipment was recovered.

The true number of enemy dead may never be known. From two hours of constant battle, it is estimated that the enemy could have lost upward to a hundred wounded and dead, and more likely much higher. 100 families in North and South Vietnam would mourn the loss of a loved one within the next few months when the news would finally filter to them. War is not only about those who win and those who die in battle. It is also about the wives, mothers, fathers, and siblings who will never see their loved ones again. Whose hearts are broken by the news of their tragic loss. This is where the politicians need to pay attention to. History only remembers the victorious, and the fallen. Never those who endure the loss at home. These are as damaged wounded warriors as the soldiers themselves.

The years following, as each man heals the anger, feels more empathy and when remembers those desperate hours of intense combat, most would fervently honour the incredible courage of those young Vietnamese soldiers who laid down their lives for the defence of their country. The same courage of our own who risked everything on that day. Who looked death in the face, swallowed their fear at huge consequences of their psychological health, and did their duty! We will remember them. We will indeed remember them.

14

CORDON AND SEARCH

The next day, V company moved to firebase Anderson. On re-joining the company there, a week later, a part of me felt disappointed that I had missed the really 'big one', that had proved to be the largest battle in which New Zealanders had fought in since The Second World War. But, under my physical and mental state, could well have pushed my trauma over the edge, whatever that edge was.

My friends were tired from the unrelenting action and pleased to see me. Several spoke about the battle, but most sat silent, looking vacantly into space or with eyes closed. Others played cards, preferring to say little about it. Clearly, many of these once young men, who now looked old and haggard, had undergone a great deal of mental punishment.

A directive was circulated, admonishing the action of two of our men for stringing up several VC corpses by the neck as a warning. Headquarters was not impressed, and nor was I. Yet, I could understand how some of our guys, seeking to relieve the tension, could resort to such hideous behaviour. Then again, every aspect of war is equally hideous.

As soon as I arrived, my first question to them.

"Who was killed in the company? No one seems to know back in Nui Dat."

"Well, you know Des was killed the day before you were cassavaked out (casualty taken out by dust off). Then on the day before the battle, Ellwood, you know the gunner from 161 who was attached to us for a few days at the beginning of the operation."

I stood there, not wanting to believe what I was hearing.

"What happened?" I lamely asked.

"Company HQ section, where the boss was (Maj. Worsnop) and

Ellwood were walked into an enemy ambush, and Ellwood was killed. We nearly lost several signalmen and the boss, who had two VC rounds through his pack, barely missed him."

I walked away feeling nothing, while choking back a mixture of so many feelings, like having my heart ripped out, lay just below the surface demanding to be expressed. In such a short space of time, I'd let myself get close to someone, only to have them suddenly taken out of my life. I would not make that '*mistake*' again with any of these guys. A conclusion that had devastating effects of being emotionally unavailable with my future wife and children.

The company was rested for a few days, while it protected the Eastern side of Anderson. I remembered the anxiety I had suffered the last time I was here nearly two weeks earlier. I preferred to dwell on that rather than on the memory of Stuart. The large enemy unit who had attacked nearby wiping out the ARVN battalion had disappeared and therefore the threat of their return was ever present.

On February 14, travelling in APCs (armoured personnel carriers) we escorted a large truck convoy mainly filled with Australian troops back to Nui Dat, three hours' drive away. As the enemy controlled most of the road, we expected an ambush at every bend in the road. We passed many American units along the way. One US armoured squadron had several tanks piled high with body bags of dead Americans. There had been a major battle in this region, with many casualties on both sides. At one point, we saw a VC unit of about platoon strength in the distance, but they were too far away to engage or pursue.

Arriving at Nui Dat unscathed, with our throats coated with the fine red dust the vehicles had kicked that up, got washed down with a cold beer later that afternoon.

* * *

'I love ham and lima beans.'

During operations, they mostly supplied us with Australian standard field ration food-packs. They were filling, plain and mostly boring. On occasions, they supplied us with American standard issue ration packs. These were twice the size, with a greater variety of food, and we were all very pleased when they arrived. They were so big that when re-supplied, because of the weight problem with just carrying our equipment, over half of each ration pack was left piled up beside the helicopter drop after we had carefully taken our favourite cuisine. Rather than put the unused rations back on a returning Huey, they were simply blown up to prevent them from falling into enemy hands. Such an appalling waste annoyed most New Zealand troops who were brought up with parents from the great depression of the 1930s, where such waste was unacceptable.

The most detested food in the Australian field ration pack was the tin of ham and lima beans. Most food packs had one and few could eat it. It seemed that they had prepared it to make it as disgusting as possible with a specific, unsavoury taste. During the battle on February the 7th, one of the guys got slightly wounded by a stray bullet that hit him in the back. He had put on his pack for extra protection from the shrapnel and the bullet passed through his pack, and penetrated a tin of ham and lima beans. The can exploded inside his pack, depositing its contents throughout his sleeping gear and change of clothing. But it saved his life by absorbing the main thrust of the bullet that ended up in his back as a mere scratch, thanks to the can of ham and lima beans.

When he got back to Nui Dat, he nailed the shattered and carefully cleaned can to the notice board inside the mess tent, with a sign beneath saying:

'I love ham and lima beans.' It brought a chuckle to everyone at the next meal.

At the conclusion of Operation Coburg by the Australian Task Force (ATF) of which we were a part, our losses were seven dead and thirty-five wounded. This low number surprised me considering the savagery and high degree of combat the Task Force had endured.

The ATF commander received the following message from General Weyand, the American commander directing all US and Allied forces in 111 Corps area:

"Upon the termination of Operation Coburg, please accept my commendation and appreciation for the exceptional performance of the 1st ATF in defeating the enemy's TET offensive attacks against the critically important Bien Hoa – Long Binh complex. The action of discovering the movement of the 274 and 275 Regiments into their attack positions, the subsequent disruption of their attacks and the way-laying of the enemy forces as they withdrew were key factors in his defeat and reflect great credit upon the officers and men of your fine command; well done."

Observers will argue that the aftermath of Tet was that the war was all but over. Barely a Communist unit in the field was capable of sustained combat. The VC would never again be the effective fighting force it had once been, leaving the brunt of the continuing years of struggle to the North

Vietnamese Army. Had the Allies known the actual state of the enemy, bold decisions might well have spelt the end of the ground war in their favour, probably within 6 months.

However, this contention is debatable, because during the following three months, the Communists poured massive reinforcements from the north into the south. All decimated NVA units regrouped and rested. Then, on May 5, 1968, the NVA launched a series of attacks throughout the country with its main thrust on Saigon. By May 13, the Communist were driven out of the Capital, leaving 5270 dead; in contrast, the Americans lost 154 of their own men and 326 ARVN. Two weeks later, the enemy was back again in strength, this time supported by Viet Cong units, and the Allies had to start the struggle of clearing them out all over again. This development was to set a pattern for the coming years. Whenever the Communists seemed finished, invariably they recovered within months and came back as strong as ever.

February 15 was used to refit the entire company with new clothes equipment, as the local laundry had fallen to a VC attack during Tet and all uniforms in being cleaned had been destroyed. I cancelled my earlier decision to extend my tour of duty in Vietnam. I was over being a soldier and just wanted to go home.

All scheduled leave had been cancelled because of the new developments in the war. I had planned to go to Saigon for six days in March, which had been allocated months earlier. It was no longer possible, and I could only shrug off the disappointment at the price of the draw on given leave dates. Paul Hunter, our section commander, had managed to get a leave in Saigon a month before the Tet offensive, and told us of his experience there.

"I was drinking in this bar, and this big Yank, half drunk, comes over to me and tells me that no '*niggers*' are allowed in here. I could have told him I was Māori, but I'm sure it wouldn't have made any difference, so I just ignored the ignorant prick, and he went away. A little while later, he came back and kicked the bloody chair out from under me. I stood up, just about to punch him, when he pulled this f_ckin' knife out of his pocket and threatened me with it. I was so bloody mad I picked up a wine bottle from the table next to mine, smashed the bottom off and threatened the jagged glass at him, telling him to come on. All he did was to put the knife back in his pocket, turn around and walk smartly out of the bar."

"Say Paul," I asked, "what if he'd kept coming at you?"

"I would have put the broken bottle in my pocket and walked out just as smartly." We all laughed. Knowing Paul, being ex SAS, that American was truly fortunate to have taken the action he did.

That afternoon I visited several of our boys in a makeshift hospital from recently erected tents, who had been wounded in the last operation. I was surprised to see three of whom I had not realised had been wounded or fallen ill. I asked one of them what he was doing there, and he gave me a strange look. "Didn't you hear about some of us getting jungle sores where it mostly counts?"

"What do you mean?"

"Sas, you're pretty slow sometimes. You know the conditions we were under in the last month? They were bloody terrible. A bunch of us got infections under the foreskin of our 'how's your father,' and they brought us out to be circumcised." He grinned and leaned closer to me.

"Don't tell anyone, but I've found a way to stay here longer. They've been giving these tablets that are supposed to prevent us having an erection, so that our pricks will have a chance to heal. Well, I haven't taken them, and I've had an erection each morning. It bloody hurts, but it's damn well worth it to have a rest from Charlie for a while. But I think they're starting to catch on to what I'm doing, so I might be joining you blokes in about a week or so."

I smiled. "Well, I guess that beats getting dysentery."

The next day was the 16th, and we were moved by truck to help in Operation Oakleigh, a cordon and search of the village of Hoa Long, two kilometres south of Nui Dat. Despite its proximity to our home base, VC activity around this village had always been prominent and was pro-Communist. It was believed that up to forty VC were hiding or living there.

About five Australian infantry companies, other support detachments, and local Vietnamese police units put a cordon around the village. The entire population was moved to a screening area to have their personal documents checked, while we, with B company, completed a thorough sweep and house by house search. Our checking the mainly thatched small houses gave us a good idea of how the Vietnamese people lived. Even though many of these locals hated us, I felt sorry for them that we were going through all their personal belongings. Such an intrusion of their privacy must have made them hate us even more. I respected as much as possible their belongings in my search, by neatly putting their personal effects back as I found them. The main aim was to look for documents with a red star at the top, indicating military orders, as well as secret passages under fireplaces, hidden weapons behind false wall panels, and other hiding places. We worked in pairs, one man searching while the other covered him in case we found an armed VC in hiding.

Over the two days of the operation, there were several skirmishes with individual VCs that had evaded the screening process and then tried to break out of the cordon. V Company captured two VC, both wounded from a short but heated gunfire exchange. B company suffered one killed and several wounded from similar encounters. The overall results were nine VC killed, four VC and twenty-five Communist agents captured, along with forty-one VC suspects and twelve Vietnamese draft dodgers detained. By midday on the 17th, we had completed the operation and returned to Nui Dat in APC's; I didn't feel good about this latest operation.

We were now regarded as seasoned combat veterans. Major Worsnop assembled the company for a briefing and a pep-talk. As he spoke, I briefly reflected on the performance of this man. He had commanded the SAS squadron in New Zealand nine years earlier with an impressive record. He kept his distance from his men at the platoon level, though, which I took to be as shyness. But he was courageous in battle, an excellent leader, particularly during the worst of the fighting, and was responsible for our own low number of casualties. His refusal to leave any man behind when our helicopter did not show up was what impressed me the most. He concluded his briefing by telling us that we had probably seen more action than any New Zealanders since World War Two.

They were stirring words, but some of us were questioning what we were doing here. I was no longer sure if we were even on the 'right side' of honour and righteousness? Was the American belief in the domino theory really true? The then popular American propaganda that said: if Vietnam falls to communism, so will the rest of the world. A theory that would be proved untrue in 1975 when North Vietnam eventually won the war. Were the Vietnamese people fighting for the spread of communism, or simply for their liberty from local governmental corruption and international dominance? Of course, none of us then knew such answers or even such questions to ask, but for some of us, our feelings were already telling us something different to what we were being told. Despite my concerns for the purpose of being here in Vietnam, being a professional soldier meant that I was here to do a job.

Back in my tent, contemplating my thoughts provoked by the Major's speech. I could see that I was living in two distinct realities. The intellectual one of questioning. 'What's it all about?' Here were the concepts, ideologies and the justification for being here?' I noticed in this world were the judgments for and against and was starting to see that this is where anger comes from.

The other world of emotionality. I sensed that this was the one that offered more truthfulness. Feelings always told the truth about the here and now, where concepts depended on what propaganda you believed in. That feelings were more about living in the here and now, and it made more sense. Yes, I could see where I can be easily carried away by a feeling like anger, but it was dawning on me that perhaps every feeling starts with a thought from the intellect, as a judgment. Years later, I would prove this to be true, which would become a significant role in my future healing.

Thinking about feelings, I noticed that fear was decreasing with each enemy contact. That my fear response – the time between the first shot being fired and the instant of feeling in charge of my fear was shortening with each consecutive battle. Am I becoming battle hardened, or simply more suppressed in my feelings? I picked up my diary and wrote: 'In war, emotion is a sign of weakness. Or is it the way to hold on to my humanness?'

I looked at what I'd just written, which stirred more thoughts. The only way to emotionally survive combat is not to feel anything. One way to do this is by de-humanizing the enemy. To remove all feelings from taking an enemy's life. That is why, over a beer in the bar between operations, it was easy to make fun and ridicule them. They are not people. They are just a '*thing*.' But if we could not dehumanize them, and see them as actual people with feelings, dreams, their love of beauty, of children, wives, husbands, Grandparents, and friends. Would we be so willing to take part in the killing ritual of organised combat? If so, it would signal how damaged and distant we were from our own humanity.

I glanced at my already read mail that had arrived earlier that day as a distraction from my crazy thoughts. I enjoyed receiving letters, especially from my parents. I picked up a letter from Patsy, my New Zealand girl friend of whom I was very fond, and re-read it for the third time. But this time, halfway through the second page, I put it down, feeling depressed. It was too hard reading the beautiful words she had written about her feelings towards me. We had not seen each other for fifteen months, but what she wrote only encouraged me to feel love, peace, and joy. I found my reaction disturbing, for I knew such emotions would soften me and draw me back into my humanness. I concluded at that moment such feelings could lead to my getting killed or going crazy. I wrote a letter back to her, breaking off the relationship and all further contact. As I finished writing, my depression lifted, and I lay on my bed, drifting back into the futile activity of thinking.

I noticed that the married men amongst us were finding the tour much more difficult. I guess they had more to live for back home but being single gave me no such distractions. Several married guys had already been sent back to New Zealand as psychologically unfit for further combat. (In the Second World War, it was called 'shell shock'). I had some judgments towards them, but years later realised that they were the true heroes. After all, they had the courage to feel their emotions while I was busy escaping mine. Torn between the love of their wives, children and doing their duty with orders to kill fellow human beings and staying alive must have been almost impossible. Was it really heroic to charge towards the enemy in a contact, not feeling anything? Perhaps it was more heroic to act while feeling one's fear than acting with one's feelings completely closed? Perhaps, just a little perhaps – "If you have never felt your fear, have you really felt your courage?"

Then I remembered when I totally felt my fear in my worst moments and my whole reality changed with everything slowing down and me feeling amazingly happy. Was I feeling my courage or was I going insane? This thought and the feelings associated would resurface in my future healing, but in this moment, I concluded the experience was a sign that I was losing my sanity.

My thoughts drifted to the action of killing. Were there exceptions to the commandment, 'Thou shalt not kill?' If there were exceptions, were they not justifications for revenge or to control people through threats and rules, which are essentially through fear? And who was to decide what the exceptions were, anyway? Is anyone wise enough to make such a decision?

I reached the point where I could no longer cope with my confusion. Getting up from my bed, I headed towards the Australian HQ lines, where I knew Father Burke was, and found him in his tent with little trouble.

After thanking him for giving up his ride for me at Anderson, and talking about the state of the war, our conversation moved on to deeper issues. I found his words comforting, even inspiring, and he put some issues to rest for me. But in other points, it only deepened my confusion, particularly around the 'Thou shalt not kill' issue. In that moment, despite the obvious contradictions, it seemed that in my job as a soldier, the exceptions were little more than justifications designed to make me '*feel better*.'

But for now, my confusion proved to be a wonderful gift, as it became a deep curiosity and, from that point, I decided to search into the deeper spiritual aspect within myself. I sensed my emotions were a key and perhaps I will experiment with them in the next contact with the VC, if I am able.

I left Father Burke and returned to my tent, realizing that religious doctrine was not enough for me anymore. Feeling inspired with a new determination to discover what made the universe tick and my relationship to it. Right now, I still have to survive the rest of my tour as an infantry soldier, and that is going to involve doing things that one day, hopefully, I may understand.

Over the next twenty years, my enquiries were to take me on the most exciting inner journey. A journey that started with the help of a wonderful priest, who probably didn't realize or intend to inspire me to take responsibility for my own spiritual life. But more importantly, of questioning my reality in the craziest time in my life, in that tent in a land far away.

My physical strength was returning, and I could go for a run each day whilst in Nui Dat. Believing myself to be cured of dysentery, I decided not to bother to check in at the hospital when I returned to Malaysia. This unwise decision was to nearly cost me my life, for the relapse of the symptoms that followed months later was worse than the original condition.

Those three days in Nui Dat before the next operation gave us time to rest, write letters, play cards, and have a few beers. The day before the next operation, Graham, Andy and I walked over to the American 183rd Artillery Battery that housed the massive 175mm guns, two kilometres away from our lines. They had the largest artillery pieces I had ever seen. The shells were so large that a crane attached to each gun loaded them. In the following months, we were to see the enormous craters made by these gigantic weapons.

The Americans treated us like royalty. We were a novelty for them, and they fed and kept supplying us with an endless stream of beer until we could barely stand. We staggered home later that afternoon, singing all the dirtiest songs that we could remember at the tops of our voices. As we passed an Australian Company Headquarters, one of their officers ran out, shouting for us to come to attention. The three of us stopped and looked at him. Then looked at each other and burst out laughing, whilst hurling insults in Malay in his direction. He called out again and started walking briskly toward us.

'Oh, what a tiresome person this is, who actually believes he can control us.' Pointing our rifles at him and shouted, "Bang, bang, you're dead, f_ck off," at which Andy cautioned us, being less intoxicated, that we could be arrested, which made Graham and myself laugh even louder. At that point, the officer must have spotted Andy's green New Zealand beret, for he at once turned around and disappeared back into his office. A wise choice, than dealing with three drunken New Zealand soldiers, carrying high velocity semi-automatic weapons. Probably for us as well, as in our drunken stupor, we may have done something we would regret for the rest of our lives.

Every night in Nui Dat, an incessant barrage of artillery fire disturbed our sleep, reminding us that the war continued to grind on. At least every hour, an infantry group in the field was in enemy contact, activating the artillery fire support.

On February 20, we left our base by truck for the next mission, 'Operation Clayton', another 'cordon and search', at the village of Long Dien. This time we were part of the cordon, but on the second day we helped with the search alongside troops of 7 RAR (Royal Australian Regiment) a fine battalion, also based at Nui Dat, that had accompanied us and 2 RAR throughout most of our previous operations.

On this occasion, we made no contact with any VC, an unusual and welcome occurrence. But in our search, we found large quantities of medical equipment destined for VC units operating in the area. The five thousand Vietnamese living in the village were screened, which resulted in the detention of forty-five draft dodgers, twelve ARVN soldier deserters, and Thirty VC suspects.

In the late afternoon, helicopters transported us back to Nui Dat. One carrying Australian troops crashed, probably as the result of enemy sniper ground fire, but miraculously there were no serious casualties.

The rubber trees around our tents were becoming quite a hazard, as three fell over in one day and a further twenty that looked threatening were cut down.

The next few days were spent patrolling at platoon strength in the jungle and scattered bush surrounding Nui Dat. Apart from seeing a lone VC in the distance who quickly disappeared, and blowing up several unexploded bombs and shells that we found, this period was happily uneventful.

Early in the morning of February 27, whilst we were lying in ambush just before 'stand to,' a large battle erupted in the direction of Long Dien, several kilometres from our position. Apparently, the VC had attacked the police station there and overrun much of the village, killing most of the ARVN. At 8 a.m. we were recalled to Nui Dat, quickly re-rationed, and in mid-afternoon were on our way by helicopters to retake Long Dien.

Before leaving, I was re-positioned as cover scout with Bill Taare. Laden with extra hand grenades for street fighting, we were set down in a dried paddy field a short distance from the village. After clearing the choppers, our section, with Bill and I leading, set off on foot towards the village.

On the outskirts of the village, was scattered bush and some thick jungle. As Bill entered this undergrowth, I noticed that he, in my opinion, was not taking the best route. I hissed at him to catch his attention. Glancing carefully to his front and flanks to secure our safety, he slowly retreated to where I was crouched on the ground and kneeled beside me. I asked:

"Why are you going right? If you go left, the going is easier for us and the rest of the Platoon following." I whispered. A brief flicker of annoyance crossed his face. Then he sighed and softened, as if to be patient with me.

"I know you received your bush training with SAS and if we go your 'left' way, it will be easier going, but it offers less cover. If we meet Charlie, we are going to need all the cover we can find, okay?"

I sort of knew this already and nodded my agreement. This valuable reminder was to later save my life when confronted by a VC master-bushman. We would stalk each other for nearly 30 minutes to get that winning shot. My whole life was to suddenly change in those future desperate moments.

* * *

As we became clear of the jungle and approached the village, Bill looked back at me and sent me a friendly wink. I smiled back at our mutual understanding.

Because they had not cleared the population out as in the earlier cordon and search operation, high Command was concerned for the safety of the locals. Thus, we had new orders of engagement, only to fire if first fired upon. Bill and I agreed, through whispers, that if we meet a local carrying a weapon, we will not wait to be fired upon.

As we entered the village, there was an uneasy hush. There were no signs of the enemy and in the distance, we could see the locals going about their business, but as they caught sight of us approaching, they became alarmed and quickly disappeared into their huts.

Once in the village, we were put into pairs to search and spread out. If the door was closed as most of them were, one man would kick open the flimsy bamboo door of a hut and leap in, weapon at the ready, while the other would cover him.

Some villagers were frightened and sat on the floor as we searched their houses. Others simply smiled. I was thankful that the VC had pulled out just before our arrival, as many civilians would have been hurt or killed in the crossfire of any fire fight. Mostly, the locals were cooperative, but it was obvious who supported the Viet Cong as they would stare at us coldly. Every house had to be searched for any possible VC hiding there, or for hidden weapons. As before, I felt sorry for the many families who had to be subjected to their invasion of privacy by foreign soldiers, mostly unaware of their customs of respect. The Māori's among us tended to be more sensitive on this issue.

As we progressed with no unwelcomed discoveries, we felt more at ease and perhaps too relaxed. Whilst Bill was searching one room, I wandered off by myself into the next hut. The door was partly open, and I walked inside. Two old Vietnamese gentlemen sitting at a table stood up as I entered. Smiling and talking excitedly, both approached me from different sides of the table. I instantly recognised the danger as they may be VC feigning friendship.

"Dung lai" ('halt' in Vietnamese) I said, pointing my rifle in their direction. But they either did not understand my accent, or refused to obey, and continued approaching from two different directions. Further alarmed, I fingered the safety catch on my rifle to ensure it was ready to fire.

"Dung lai!" I said firmly and shook my rifle menacingly at the nearest one. They kept coming, smiling and unaware of my rising panic. Taking the first pressure on my trigger in readiness to fire, I thrust my rifle muzzle menacingly towards the closest one and yelled, "Dung bloody lai." He staggered back and raised his hands above his head, looking frightened as they both finally understood that I meant business. I motioned with my rifle that they stand in the corner of the room where I could easily watch them. Keeping my rifle trained in their direction, I quickly inspected the room. It was clear, and I realised they were only being friendly. The old man I confronted may never know how close to death he came on that day. I would have certainly fired had he taken one more step. I walked out to look for Bill, aware of my foolishness of having departed from the standard searching procedure.

Throughout the village, there was much evidence of heavy fighting in the early morning battle, and many buildings had been destroyed. It was unclear how many civilians had become casualties. After completing the search, we reassembled and returned to the dried paddy field where we dug in for the night.

The next morning, we moved back into the village for another quick search and after that, sat down along the street, resting against the huts, waiting for further orders. Soon, the locals appeared from their houses and talked to us. The atmosphere had changed from the fear and suspicion of the previous day to one of friendliness. This was the first real social contact we'd made with the local Vietnamese people. An old gentleman came over to us and gave me a soft drink and I thanked him in Vietnamese. A young woman standing at his side echoed my thanks back in English. I smiled at her and was struck by her beauty.

Young children ran about, and we gave them sweets and biscuits, but I couldn't take my eyes off this radiant young Vietnamese woman. Though her English was limited, we managed to hold a simple conversation. Not having been close to a woman for such a long time, I found my attraction quickly rising. However, I felt awkward and unsure of what to say next, and often referred to my Vietnamese phrase-book supplied by the Americans. A feeling of mutual attraction seemed to flow between us as we fumbled over our conversation. Our awkwardness increased our attraction to one another, perhaps because we were being real with a touch of vulnerability to each other.

"Okay, saddle up and let's move out." The sharp command from Sgt. John Whitworth brought our all too brief idyll to an abrupt end.

As we moved out, her older companion, whom I assumed was her father, rushed over to me and handed me a large bag of fruit, with her smiling on. His torrent of Vietnamese was beyond my comprehension, but he was clearly bidding me farewell and good fortune, which was very touching. The thought of that woman tortured me for days afterwards.

PTSD: By now, most of us were reeling from PTSD (Post Traumatic Stress Disorder) commonly known in WW2. as shellshock. Symptoms included recurring nightmares, short tempers and later the main ones were alcohol and drug addiction, domestic violence, and anti-social behaviour. Mine, which is the most common, came as a drastic loss of self-confidence, that was to plague my life for the next twenty years. It was finally healed through the practise of Breath Integration.

* * *

15
AMBUSHED

Modern day jungle warfare was not only about patrolling looking for suspected enemy locations on search and destroy operations, but also setting up ambush sites. Nearly 50% of enemy contacts were through this military tactic. They were mostly set up in a bend or a junction on a track, river crossing and roads that were used by the VC. They too used this means of combat against allied troops and we ourselves fell victim to their skilful positioning of this dreaded trap. Few ever escaped alive from a well-constructed ambush site. This was how Stuart had died.

The most feared weapon used in an ambush other than the machine gun was the claymore mine. The VC also had such a weapon, which was bigger, with more explosive and ball bearings that created so much destruction to a human body. Fortunately for us, their version was less effective because of a poor design and shape. Ours were more carefully designed to explode in a set direction, causing more confined and concentrated lethal blast areas up to 60 metres. We can only wonder that designers of such terrible weapons had to be mentally damaged, disconnected from their emotions, their humanness, and the appalling effects of their invention. We could extend this out to include all weapons or war.

The next few days we spent patrolling north, from Long Dien to the outskirts of Hoa Long. Trouble was expected, so we set up ambushes every night. As Blue Neame had stayed behind in Nui Dat, they gave me the section's M60 machine gun. It took several hours to get used to the extra weight in my hands, and I was very happy to give it back to Blue when he returned to the platoon two days later. My SLR rifle had never felt so light!

The next night, around midnight, we were shattered from our sleep by the sound of explosions and automatic gunfire only metres away. My first thought was that the ambush site had been sprung, but then I realised that the firing was behind us. The unmistakable staccato sound of several Communist AK47 assault rifles, followed by the comforting sound of our own M60 returning fire. A hail of bullets shot low overhead with their unmistakable cracking sound, stripping leaves and small branches off trees, and kicking up the ground around us. It was so dark I could see nothing, not even the enemy gunfire flashes, so refrained from firing towards the sound of the VC lest I hit any of our own guys. I pulled out my bayonet and fixed it to my rifle in case any VC came charging at us through the thick jungle, as I wouldn't see them until they would be right on top of me. This extra protection was comforting,

I lay holding my rifle in readiness and examined what I was feeling, which was excitement with elements of fear under control. I noticed something else that I had largely ignored in previous contacts and that I was hardly breathing. Then, remembering that many times during previous battles, I would hold my breath. Intuitively, I felt that this was connected to the fear response, which years later, I would prove true.

Laying in my shell scrape with my body below the ground, I knew I was reasonably safe and only the small area of my face being exposed as I peered into the darkness. It was not surprising that so many badly wounded and killed were shot through the face, being a major part of my regular nightmare. Minutes later, the firing stopped as the enemy pulled out.

A squad of VC or NVA had been moving through the scattered bush twenty metres parallel to the track on which we had laid the ambush. They had missed the ambush team and walked straight into our platoon position. As it had been so dark, our sentry and the VC squad saw each other only three steps away from each other. Both hastily opened fire and miraculously missed each other.

Minutes after the firing stopped, the entire area was bathed in bright light as mortar illumination flares from Nui Dat lit up the sky directly overhead. Suddenly, shell cases falling off the flares as they exploded in the air thudded into the ground all around us. One landed five metres from where I was lying. Made of heavy metal, they would fall from a great height and were extremely dangerous to anything or anyone they landed on. Not for the first time, I regretted not wearing an American steel helmet instead of our light cotton jungle hats. I pulled out my small folding shovel, quickly unscrewed it, and held the blade over my head, hoping to provide some protection. Several of the guys cried out in alarm and I could hear Danny McPhail on the radio talking agitatedly to the mortar crews to cease firing. It took some minutes before, to everyone's relief, they finally stopped. They were soon followed by high explosive shells that landed about 200 metres away. This experience from the falling shell cases shook us more than from the contact with the Viet Cong.

Steve came round, checking on casualties. "Is everyone all right? Blue, IB, Grease gun, Barney, are you okay?" He reached me.

"Sas?"

"Yeah, I'm fine now that our mortars have stopped dropping objects on us. Has anyone been hurt?"

"Yes, Alan Haua 'copped' it, but not from the shell cases. Charlie got him, but he was talking when I passed him a few minutes ago. I don't think it's too bad. Through the leg, I think. They're dressing the wound now."

We pulled the ambush team back into the safety of the platoon harbour in case the VC returned for another go and waited out the rest of the night with half of us on 'stand to.'

The next morning, I saw Alan sitting up, unusually white-faced for a Māori, with a blanket over his shoulder and legs.

"Where'd you get it, Alan?" I asked gently as I sat down beside him.

"A nick in the shoulder and one clean through the foot, near the ankle. They thought it better to keep my boot on and dress that, rather than try to put a dressing directly on the foot. I dunno what they'll find when they take my boot off in Nui Dat, but it doesn't hurt too much. Shoulder's just a scratch."

"Now you know it's against standing orders to shoot yourself in the foot* to get out of here," I joked. "It's better to get dysentery. It works, every time."

He smiled weakly and pointed to the M79 grenade launcher lying beside him.

"Sorry, but you'll have to take back your baby and the M16 rifle. I'm out of here later this morning. Wilson says he wants you to take it back, okay Sas?"

"Of course." I answered, picking up the M79, wiping off some of Alan's caked blood from the butt with my shirtsleeve. We exchanged weapons, ammunition, and grenades, and on standing up, felt the extra weight.

** *Shooting oneself in the foot by soldiers during the First World War to escape the fighting, became so prevalent that the military brought out serious punishments to stop it.*

"See you back in Kiwi Land. Give those girls a taste of what they can expect when I get there, you lucky bastard."

Alan nodded as I walked back to my position. He was lifted out by dust off helicopter later that morning.

It was March 1st, and we continued patrolling the general area. On one pleasant note, I noticed now how much more I lived for the moment, or perhaps for the next meal or rest stop at the most. My old habit of planning for the future, and daydreaming about next week, or next year, even though I might be dead the following week, was sliding away. I later came to recognise the value of living in the present, known in Buddhism as mindfulness. I never appreciated what a wonderful gift it was. In my diary I wrote as if it were a disorder; 'My dreams and thoughts have been reduced to this'. Despite all the horror in my daily life, there was a quality of aliveness and a sense of presence, in which there was no fear, suffering, or thoughts of how terrible everything was. Everything 'just was,' with an element of pleasure in small things. Even the boring army ration packs were a delight, as if I were eating this delicious meal for the first time. Such a joy of living in the 'now' also slid away when I went back to normal life at the end of my tour. I rediscovered this years later through meditation, breathing, and Integrative Presence. When faced with death every day, we live the day in every moment as it might be our last.

Just at dusk, we moved out towards a new ambush position two kilometres away. Twenty minutes later, as the last traces of light faded from the sky, our lead scout suddenly froze. This was the formal warning that something was wrong, and we could barely see the turned-down thumb signal being silently passed from the front man down the line. We all froze. I was sixth in line in the front section. With no command, we moved up and spread out to support our lead scouts. Before we could fully form a broad front, firing broke out from our scouts and from enemy fire. My growing experience with the M79 grenade launcher told me in a glance that a forward right flank position offered the best field of fire. Sprinting towards that direction, I passed Blue, who was standing fearlessly, legs astride, firing his M60 machine gun from the hip as if it were a toy. He might well have been a model for the future Rambo! The rest of the platoon had found cover or were on the ground returning fire.

Whilst still running, I ripped the M79 from my shoulder, and then, on reaching cover, threw myself behind a log. I slowly raised my head above my cover and saw that I was well positioned, slightly forward on the right flank of the platoon, alone. In the darkness, it was not possible to see through the sights, and so I had to judge the elevation of the weapon to fire at the enemy gun flashes about sixty metres away. I could make out the dim outline of two VC crouched on the ground behind a termite hill that dotted the landscape. Concealed from the platoon, both were concentrating their automatic fire towards them, not seeing me on their left flank. My first grenade over-shot, but my next, seconds later, exploded right on target, and the two VC disappeared. Then, from behind another termite hill close by, one VC again opened fire. He was wildly spraying his automatic fire in sweeping motions like a garden hose, now including my position. The familiar cracking sound as each round passed close overhead made my ears ring and forced us all to keep our heads down. As he emptied his magazine, it took just a few seconds to replace it and open fire again. I carefully elevated my M79, judging the most exact position, raised my head and fired, but missed. As he saw my gun flash caused him to fire back in my direction and I ducked down behind my shelter as his bullets thudded into my log. As he swept his fire back to the platoon, I peered over my cover, fired another grenade, and quickly ducked down. I wasn't sure where it landed, but his firing stopped. After a slight pause, he fired again, but his fire was more erratic and wilder, as if wounded. I fired again, and this grenade landed right on the termite hill he was sheltering behind, and he stopped firing.

I checked in to see what I was feeling. It had all taken place so quickly that there had not been time to think about the danger, and so I felt no fear, but I was holding my breath. As I took a deep breath and breathed out a sigh of relief, I noticed my hands shook, a sign that my body had experienced stress at some level. It occurred to me that perhaps there was a correlation between thinking, feeling fear, and breathing, or the holding of the breath. Something I would later prove through Breath Integration that would be a major factor in my future healing. For now, it was just a contemplation.

I could not help admiring the bravery of this VC. He had us all pinned down for the duration of the contact.

The platoon started moving up.

"Good bloody shooting, Sas," exclaimed one guy as he caught up and walked past. Hamish Wilson directed our section to sweep forward in an extended line while the rest of the platoon covered us. The tall, rounded termite hill where the two VC had disappeared behind was in a cleared area with no bush nearby, stood bare and threatening.

"If Charlie is still alive, that's where they'll fire from," I whispered to Colin Burgering, who was slowly moving forward on my left.

"Yeah, we would have seen them had they had tried to run off, so they must still be there. Shit, this is a ropey one, Sas," he whispered back.

I glanced past him and then to my right and realised most of the rest of the section was to spread out. This meant that Colin and I were isolated at the centre of the sweep and if Charlie fires, we will be the obvious targets.

"Bloody hell, move in closer to support us," I hissed into the night to the rest of the section. Either they didn't hear, or chose not to, for they kept their distance from us. I could not blame them, for who would want to make themselves an obvious target to a possibly wounded enemy waiting, with no chance of escape. At least the section should support us with return fire if Charlie has a go at us. Feeling totally exposed and vulnerable, it took all my willpower to take each step forward, thinking it might be my last. I noticed I felt intense fear and was holding my breath as I thought about the danger I was in.

As Colin and I reached the termite hill, both ready to fire at the slightest movement, Colin cautiously went to its left, and I crept around to the right. Nothing!

"Where'd they go?" he whispered. Colin crouched down, scratching his head. It was not possible for them to have vanished like that. At least there should have been dead bodies or, worse, live ones. In the dark, we could see a pool of blood on the ground beside the termite hill.

"Well, at least one of them is badly wounded," Colin further commented, just as the rest of the section caught up with us. Then they combed the area, while Colin and I acted as cover from the termite hill. Still nothing.

"I feel they are here, close by," I whispered to Colin. "They can't just disappear. They must be here somewhere."

The rest of the platoon joined us, and after one last search, we all moved on towards our ambush site, still bewildered by the disappearing VC. After travelling through knee-deep swamp, then dried paddy, we reached the road between Long Dien and Hoa Long and set up an ambush. No enemy ventured near us that night.

At first light the next morning, we returned to check the area where we had the contact the night before. After a search in daylight, we found a blood trail leading from the termite hill into the bush. Carefully checking the termite hill, we found a trap door that had been skilfully concealed on the top.

"Cunning buggers," John Linley breathed as he carefully checked the small door for booby traps with his bayonet before gently easing it open.

Inside a small room had been dug out and at the bottom lay the body of a dead VC.

"The other one must have sheltered here until we left last night and took both weapons, as wounded as he was." Blue added.

Close by, another hideout with a trap door was found, but it was empty. We called in Australian engineers who arrived by helicopter an hour later and laid explosive charges inside both hideouts. After searching the dead VC and leaving him inside, the engineers blew up the hideouts, denying the enemy their future use. As we moved out, I glanced at the mutilated remains of the corpse. All that remained was his torso, with his legs, one arm and head blown off. It was still a horrible sight, even though by this time, I had seen many dead bodies.

For the next week, we set up a series of ambushes on track junctions and roads, and then hid in the jungle during the day. However, when our ambushes brought no results, it seemed as if the back of the enemy had been broken from the Tet offensive. Hamish Wilson split the platoon and ordered Sgt. Whitworth to take one half to set ambushes away to our east. This procedure, he felt, would double our effectiveness.

As we patrolled, most of us felt on edge throughout the day for some unexplained reason. The thundering boom of 175mm guns from Nui Dat suddenly opened fire, several kilometres away, causing us all to jump with fright. The noise from these enormous guns never bothered us before. But, like a premonition, we all sensed something horrendous might happen.

Just on dusk, the night of March 6, 1968, our half of the platoon, commanded by Hamish Wilson, moved to a new area. We passed a dead water buffalo near a deserted and isolated hut in a cleared part of the jungle, with its calf standing next to it. It looked confused and bewildered why its mother would not move and feed it. The buffalo appeared to have been dead for about two days and was a pathetic sight. I forced myself to choke back any sentimental feelings.

We travelled on through scattered bush and rolling hills. Suddenly, my senses warned me of danger. All the usual evening insect sounds suddenly stopped, with an eerie silence. I wondered if Barney, our lead scout, was feeling the same, or was it just my vivid imagination?

Suddenly, the entire jungle to our immediate front and right erupted in massive gunfire and exploding claymore mines. As I hit the ground, I knew we had walked into an enemy ambush. Payback time for the dozen of VCs we had killed in our ambushes. We all returned fire from wherever we were; with no time to look for cover. We were desperate with our only hope being to win the firefight. In those first few seconds, I knew we were in trouble as Charlie had cover and probably outnumbered us as well.

For about sixty seconds, which seemed like an age, the firepower and the closeness of the exchange were an intensity from hell. I felt no fear. There was no time. Just a grim determination to fight until killed.

Unable to see them in the darkness, I kept firing grenades into their gunfire flashes a mere twenty metres away. I did not stop to think how many of us might already be dead; the only thought was to keep firing until hit. There was no let-up in the enemy fire, and I knew it was just a matter of seconds before I would leave this life and a thought trickled into my mind of 'let's get it over with as quickly and hopefully painlessly as possible.' Then I let this, and all thoughts go and was with what is in this moment. An acceptance of my death entered my mind.

This acceptance triggered the altered mental state, like the last time I had lost hope. Everything appeared to slow down, as if I were watching a slow-motion movie. Again, I could look around, reload, fire, and experience the same incredible sensation of happiness throughout my entire body. There seemed to be no sense of time or rapid motion; even the tracer bullets cracking close over my head seemed to be moving slowly. I saw an old shell crater next to where I was lying, and quickly, but in seemingly slow motion, rolled into it for extra cover.

"Oh no, I'm going insane again." I remembered how I stopped it last time and at once started thinking of the danger of being in the middle of a battle. It worked and everything sped up again to its normal pace and the familiar horror was back that I trusted more. I was a soldier again, engulfed with all the feelings of disgust, anger, and fear. I was controlling my insanity.

In the next instant, the enemy threw several smoke grenades between us, signalling their withdrawal, stopped firing, and melted away in the darkness and into the jungle behind them.

All firing stopped, and to our surprise, we had won.

One retreating VC, limping from a wound, ran in front of us and was immediately cut down by a burst from our machine gun. Another was crawling on the ground, desperately trying to escape. He was out of sight of the rest of our section. Only I could see him, and the thought came. 'How many of our guys are lying dead because of you?' This thought triggered an anger to swell up in me to turn to blind rage. I picked up my loaded grenade launcher and took aim to blow my mortal enemy to 'Kingdom Come'. 'No,' came another thought, 'too quick.' Deliberately I put the M79 down and picked up my M16 rifle and fired one shot and saw it strike his body. Then coldly and calculatedly fired again, again and again, feeling the bloodlust as strong as a sexual orgasm stir in me as each shot struck, tearing his body to threads. I kept firing, savouring each shot with a shocking, intense pleasure, until my 20-round magazine was empty. This was a pleasure distinctly different from the weird experience minutes before where I was calm and relaxed, and now I was tense, muscles straining with pain, rage, and revengeful bitterness. Such a state knows no boundaries.

I carefully reloaded and was about to fire again at the motionless grotesque heap on the ground when Barney's voice, close by, snapped me out of my psychotic state. He was yelling and pointing to fire at a termite hill where he had seen a lone VC disappear. I shook my head to snap myself back to my job in hand. My first grenade landed right on top of the hill, showering shrapnel over the other side. A high pitched, shrill voice, taut with fear, started screaming in broken English from the other side of the hill.

"Not VC. Not VC, ARVN. Not VC."

"It's a trick, kill the bastard," I heard someone close by angrily yell. I fired several more grenades towards the small hill. Several guys threw hand grenades, followed by a phosphorous grenade hoping to burn the VC out, but he kept screaming,

"Not VC. Not VC." We stopped firing. Someone yelled,

"Chew hoi! Yuh tie len, lie dia." But the soldier ignored the order to surrender and come out with his hands up. No doubt believing he would be killed. Two of our guys had quite enough. With fixed bayonets, they charged over the hill to finish him, but the lone soldier put up his hands and was spared. Hamish Wilson went forward to inspect the captive, and seconds later walked briskly back to Andy to radio a message back to HQ. As he passed me, he fiercely spat out, "F_ck, they are bloody ARVN."

We all went forward and formed an all-round defence. Steve did a check on each man for casualties. We were all amazed that not one of us had been wounded, let alone killed, in the heated exchange. It was a total miracle. We had been fortunate enough to have walked into an ambush by inexperienced ARVN who had fired too high and positioned their claymores ineffectively. If they had been seasoned VC, or NVA, we would all have surely died.

I moved over to the ARVN soldier, who was still lying on the ground, and saw that he was an ARVN officer. A bullet had passed through the left side of his pelvis, leaving a gaping hole on the other side of his body, and was losing a lot of blood. I pulled out my bayonet to cut his pants off him. His eyes widened in fear as he first looked at the bayonet in my hand, and then back at me. I put a reassuring hand on his shoulder and then cut and slipped his pants off. The moonlight gave me enough light as I dressed his terrible wounds. While I worked, he kept feeling with his hand between his legs to see if he had lost any of his vital parts. He was in enormous pain, and someone gave him a shot of morphine. On completion, I covered him with a blanket, and reassured him in broken Vietnamese that he should be okay.

Wandering over to where the remains of the man I had killed, I sat down beside his shattered body. I did not know how to feel and was full of confusion. I was no stranger to taking life, but this was an allied soldier. What made it worse was in the manner and attitude that I had killed him. I felt deep shame that was to be added to my expanding psychological container of trauma. I reached out and touched his shoulder, as a futile gesture of atonement. This caused his head to roll in my direction and in the moonlight, saw his sightless eyes make direct contact with mine, as if to curse me. I jumped back in fright, thinking he was still alive, and instantly swung my rifle round, ready to fire in a reflex action. He lay still, staring in my direction. I moved slightly to one side and let out my held breath as a relief that his eyes didn't follow my movement. Carefully I gently closed his eyes, then placed my hand on his chest, gently shook him, just to make sure. No, he was well dead, but so was a big part of me. I withdrew my hand, which was covered in his blood, and wiped it off on his trouser leg.

There seemed like a presence of him I sensed, and felt he was looking down at me, and then, slowly, it seemed to leave. The feeling was so strong, I uttered quietly, "Goodbye, I'm truly sorry."

Standing up, bewildered and shocked by what I'd done to this man. Friend or foe, it made no difference. Looking down at him, remembering the pleasure of killing him, and feeling appalled. 'What kind of monster am I turning into?' I asked myself. The answer to this question was too disturbing to contemplate. Torn between allegiance to my country and the growing awareness that to kill another human being is such a devastating act, I found my mind was disintegrating. I recognised I could not continue to function effectively as a soldier whilst I was so emotionally disturbed. With this realisation I cast out of my mind the memory of this most horrific experience. It was to be twenty years later when this gruesome experience was recalled and released from its pain.

By then, I was further relieved to discover through my research of the 'Fight/Flight/Freeze' syndrome that to feel this blood lust was a natural coping skill when extreme limits of one's mental endurance had been reached. It was the psyche's over-compensational attempt to normalise the event to survive mentally and emotionally.

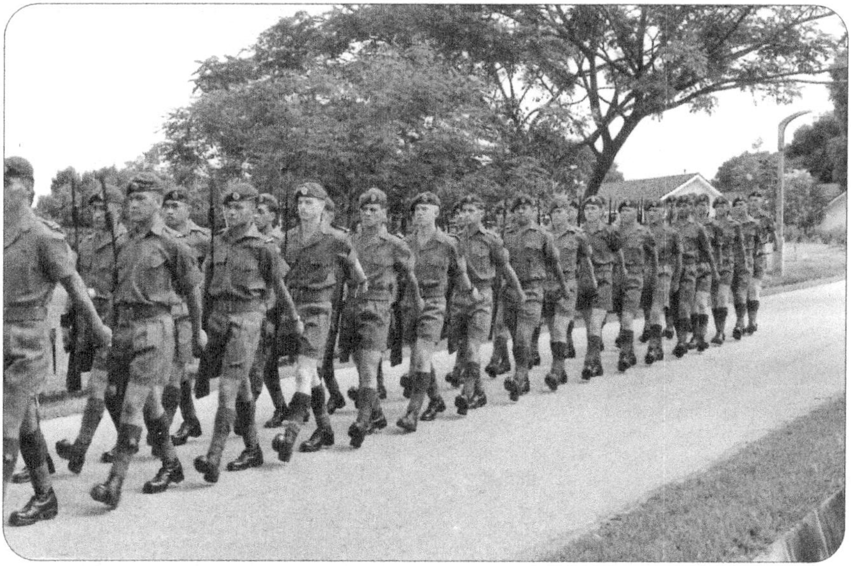

On parade in Malaysia training for Vietnam. Author 4th in closest line. Cecil Poa behind Author and John Lindley following Cecil.

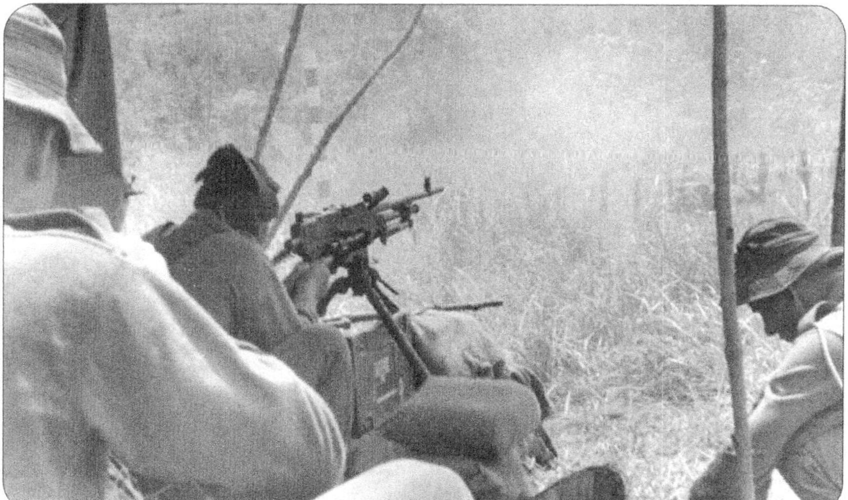

Malaysian jungle training. Crawling beneath live firing ammunition to climatize for incoming enemy fire.

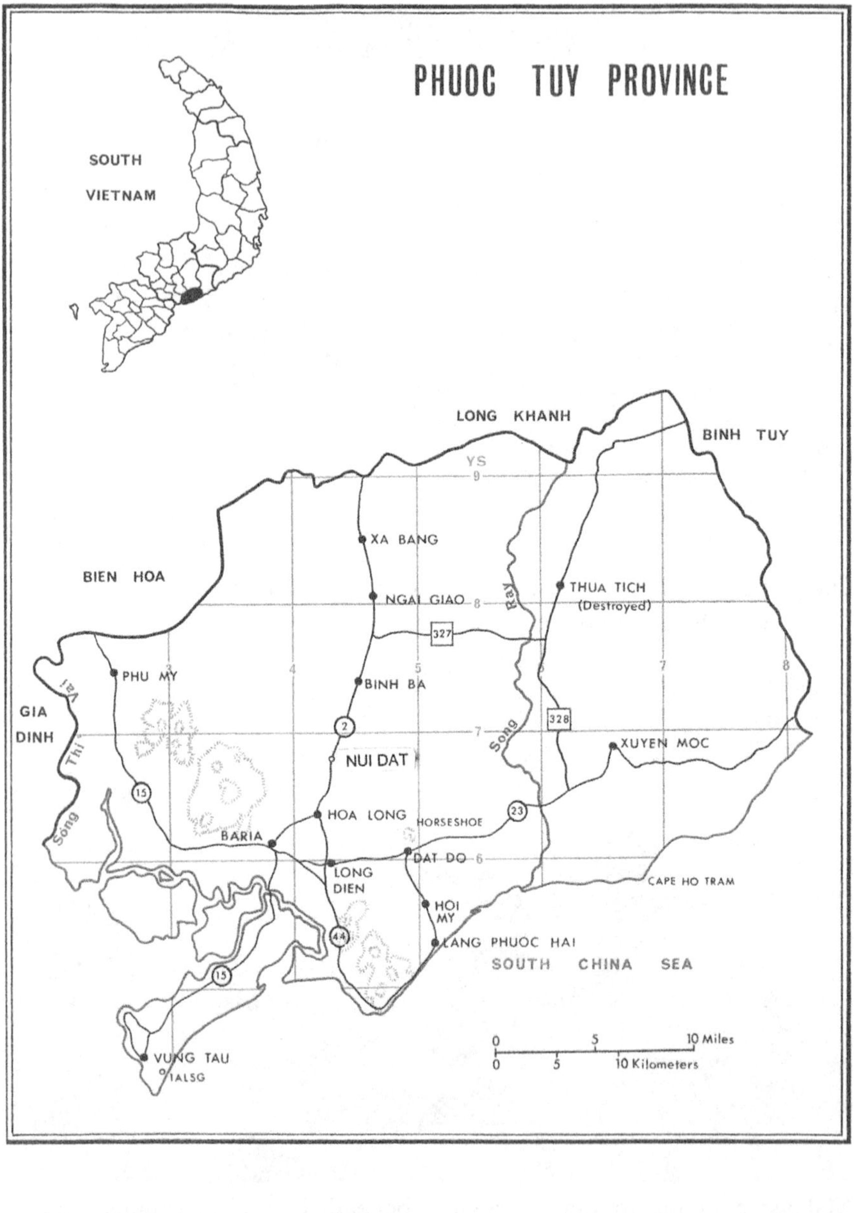
PHUOC TUY PROVINCE
SOUTH
VIETNAM
LONG KHANH
BINH TUY
BIEN HOA
GIA
DINH
XA BANG
NGAI GIAO
THUA TICH
(Destroyed)
327
PHU MY
BINH BA
328
NUI DAT
XUYEN MOC
HOA LONG
HORSESHOE
BARIA
DAT DO
LONG
DIEN
CAPE HO TRAM
HOI
MY
LANG PHUOC HAI
SOUTH CHINA SEA
VUNG TAU
1ALSG
Song Thi Vai
Song Ray
0 5 10 Miles
0 5 10 Kilometers

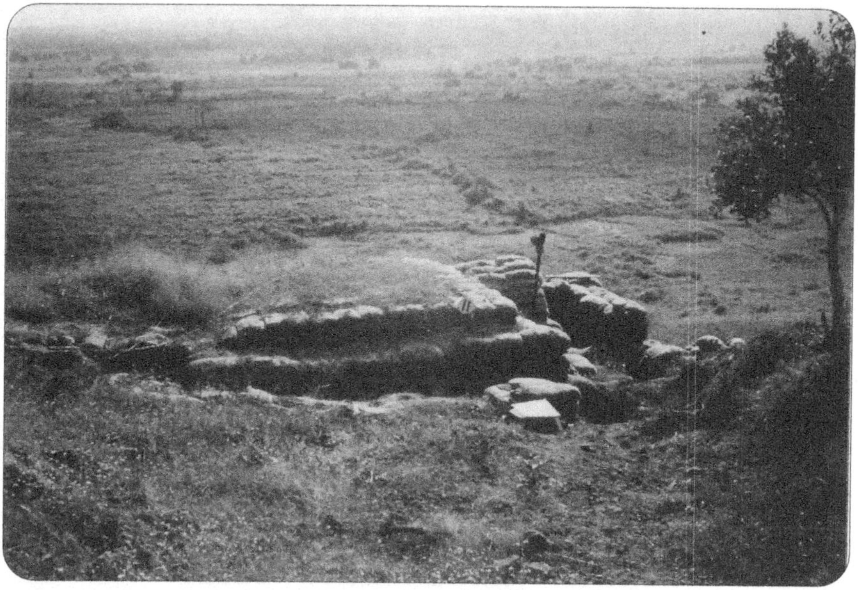

Our bunker at the Horseshoe, facing Southeast. When not on patrol, was home for six weeks. Nov. 1967

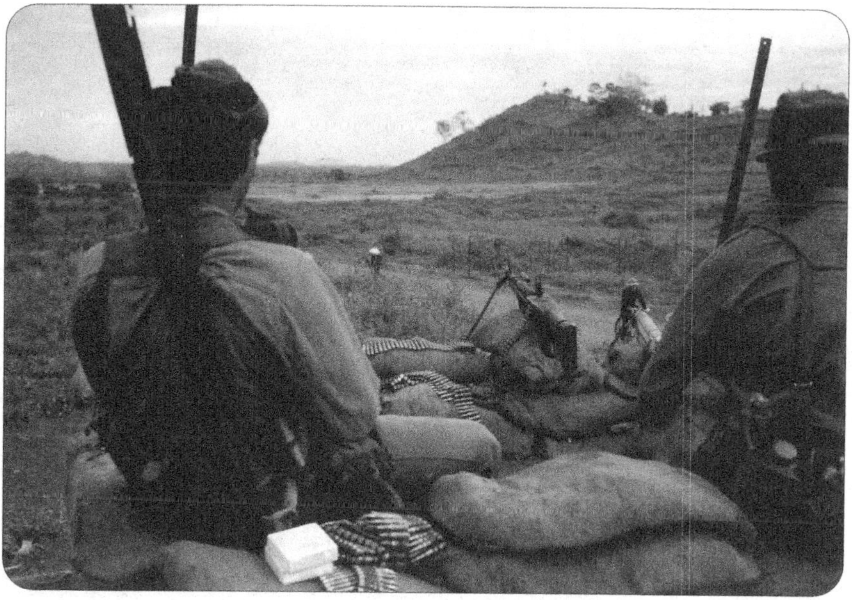

Village of Dat Do, looking towards the Horseshoe. Members of 6 Platoon manning Checkpoint Charlie. December 1967

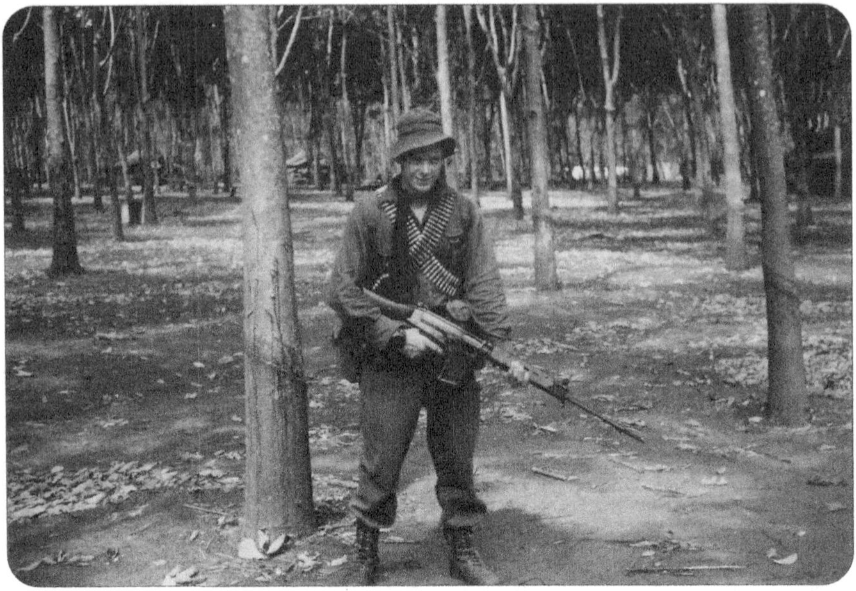

Author on the morning just before departure on Operation Duntroon. Carrying SLR (Self loading rifle) with two belts of M60 machine gun rounds that every man carried. January 1968.

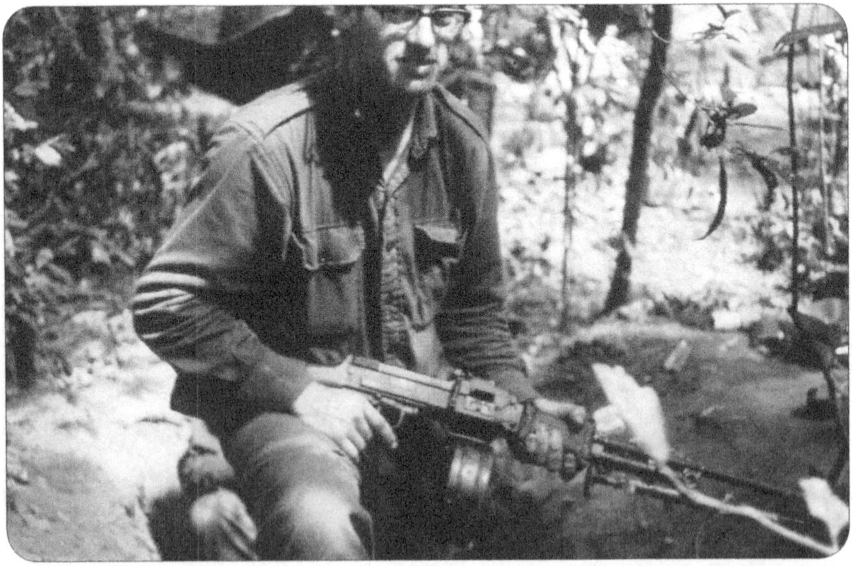

Andy Cowie holding a captured enemy Degtyaryov 7.62mm light machine gun. January 1968.

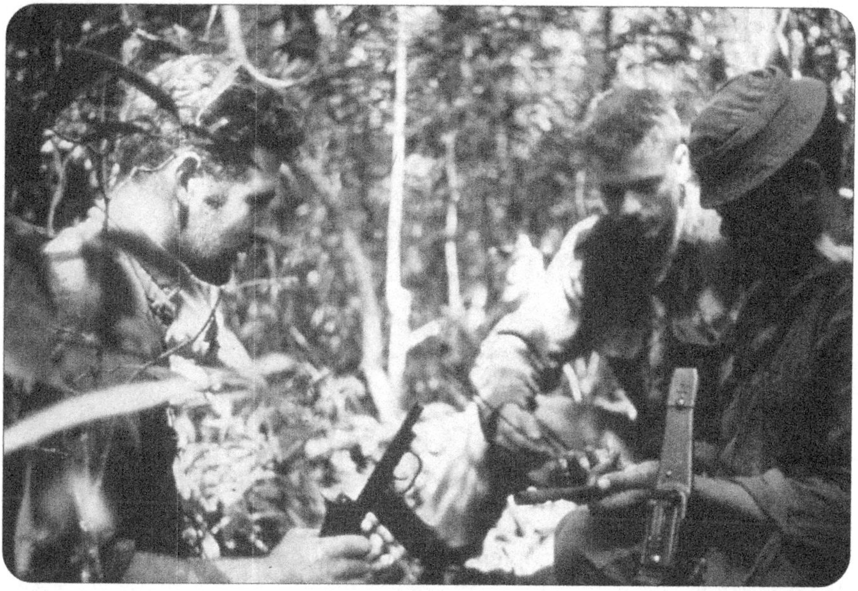

From left, Blue Neame, Author, and John Tawhara.
Operation Duntroon, January 1968.

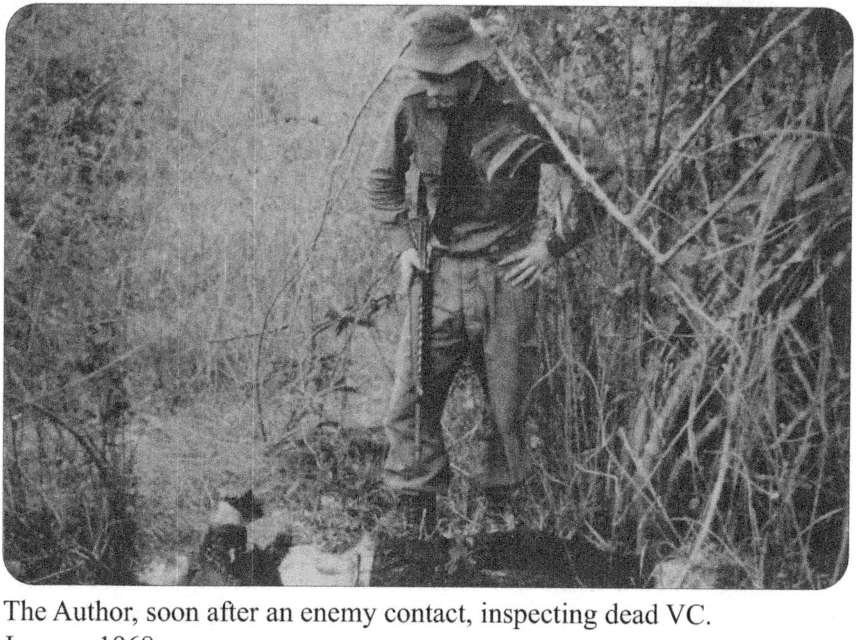

The Author, soon after an enemy contact, inspecting dead VC.
January 1968

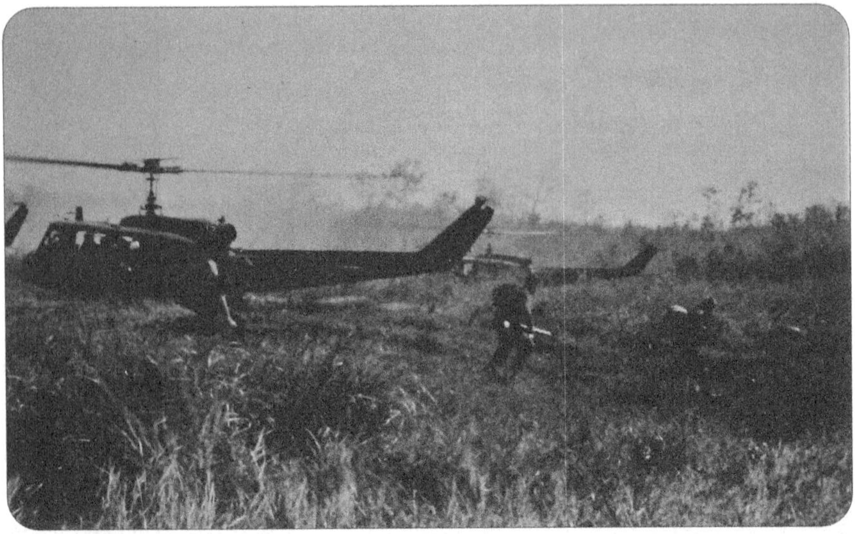

Sprinting to our 'lost' helicopter at the completion of Operation Duntroon. January 1968

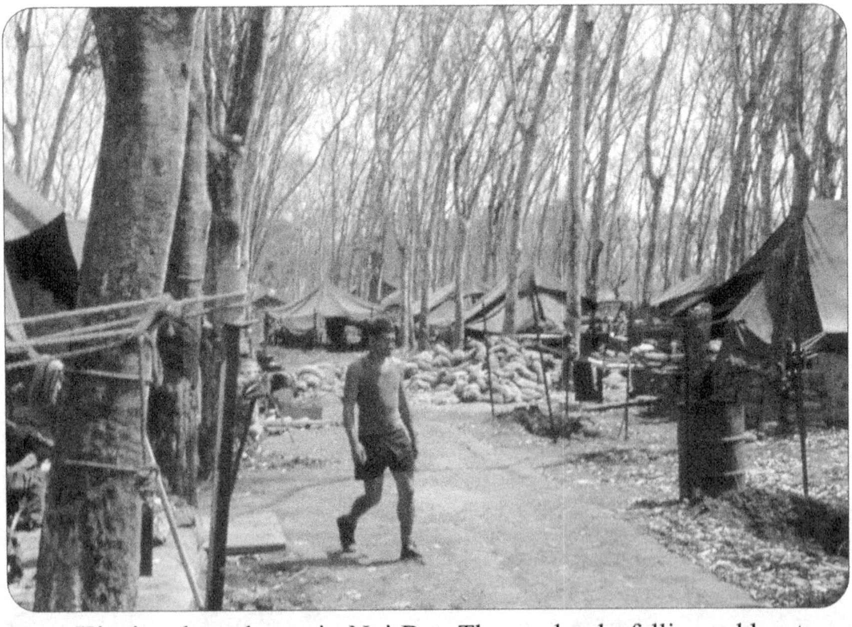

Dave Kingi and our home in Nui Dat. The randomly falling rubber trees became a serious safety problem, while here between operations.

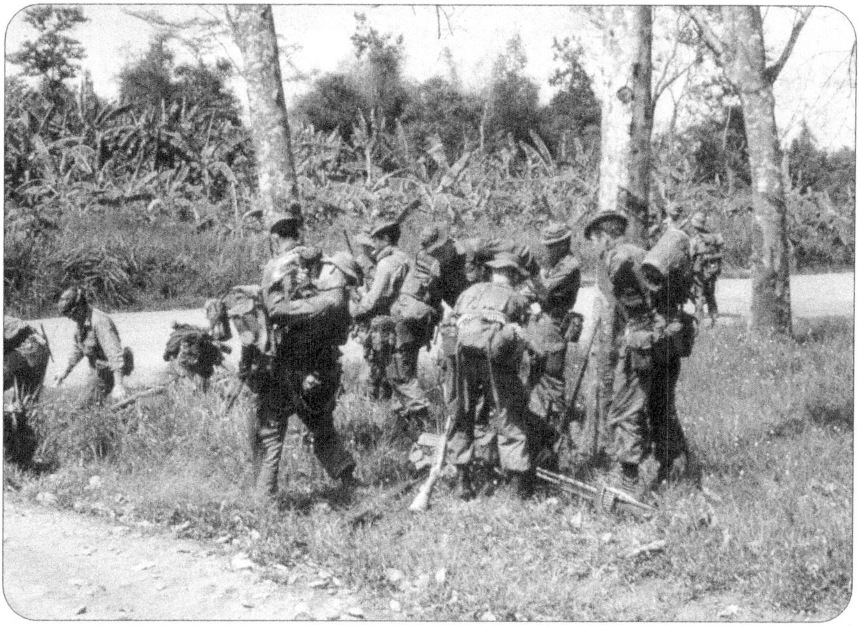

Six Platoon preparing for departure from Nui Dat on Operation Coburg, January 24th, 1968.

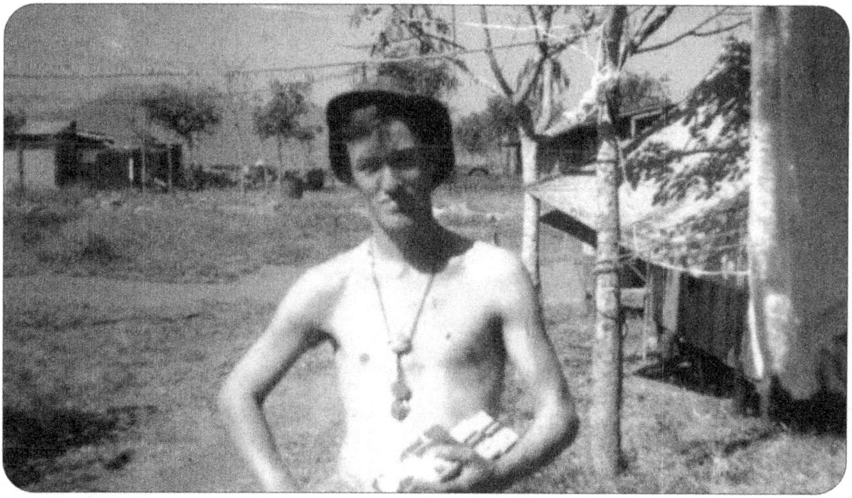

Stuart Ellwood

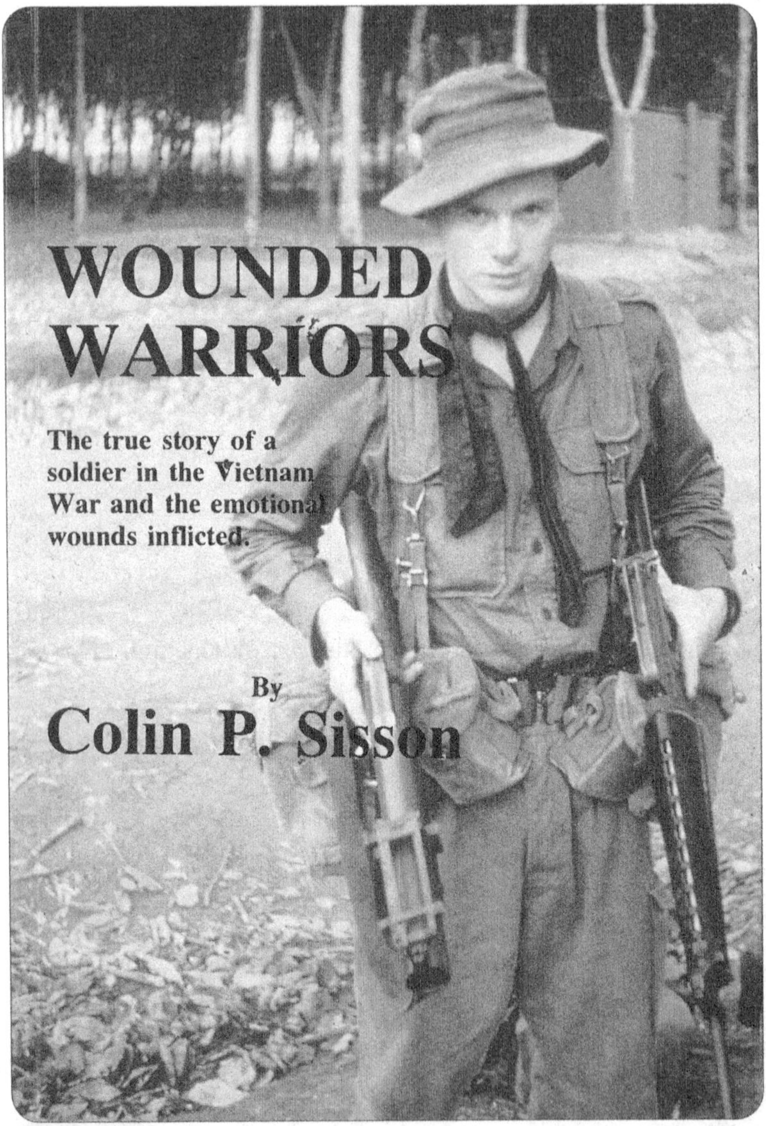

Original First Edition cover *Wounded Warriors*, Pub. 1993
Nui Dat after operation Coburg, February 1968.
In my right hand, M79 grenade launcher, other hand M16.
This was the best smile I could muster after the death of Stuart Ellwood and Des Hirini.

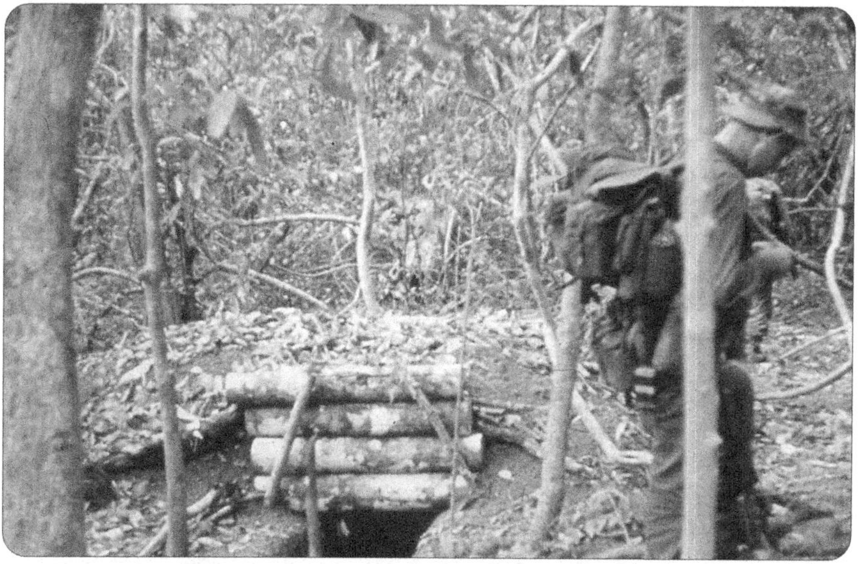

I B Paterson passing a VC bunker having just been cleared of enemy in the captured Communist camp. 1st February 1968

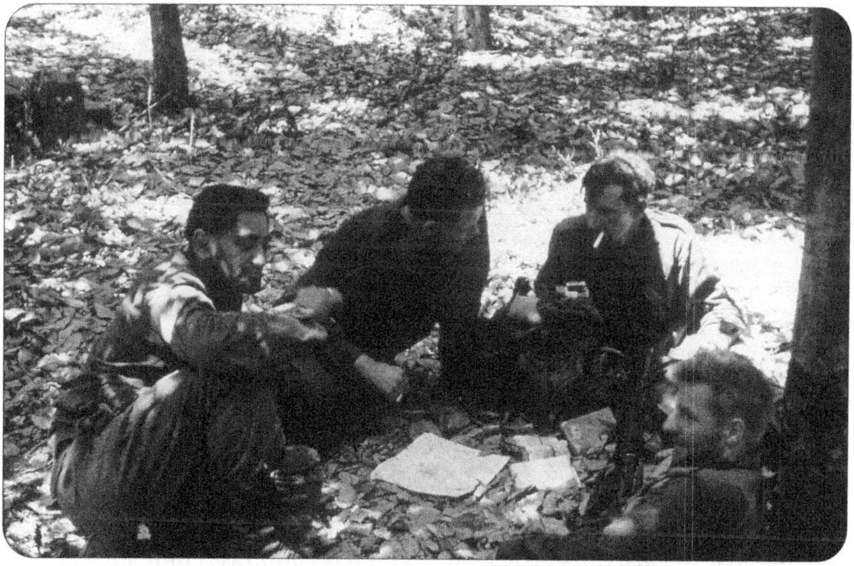

Section commanders and Platoon Sergeant. From left: Paul Hunter, Steve Vautier, Sgt. John Whitworth, Tom Whitaker. February 1968.

Major Brian Worsnop, company commander giving orders during operation

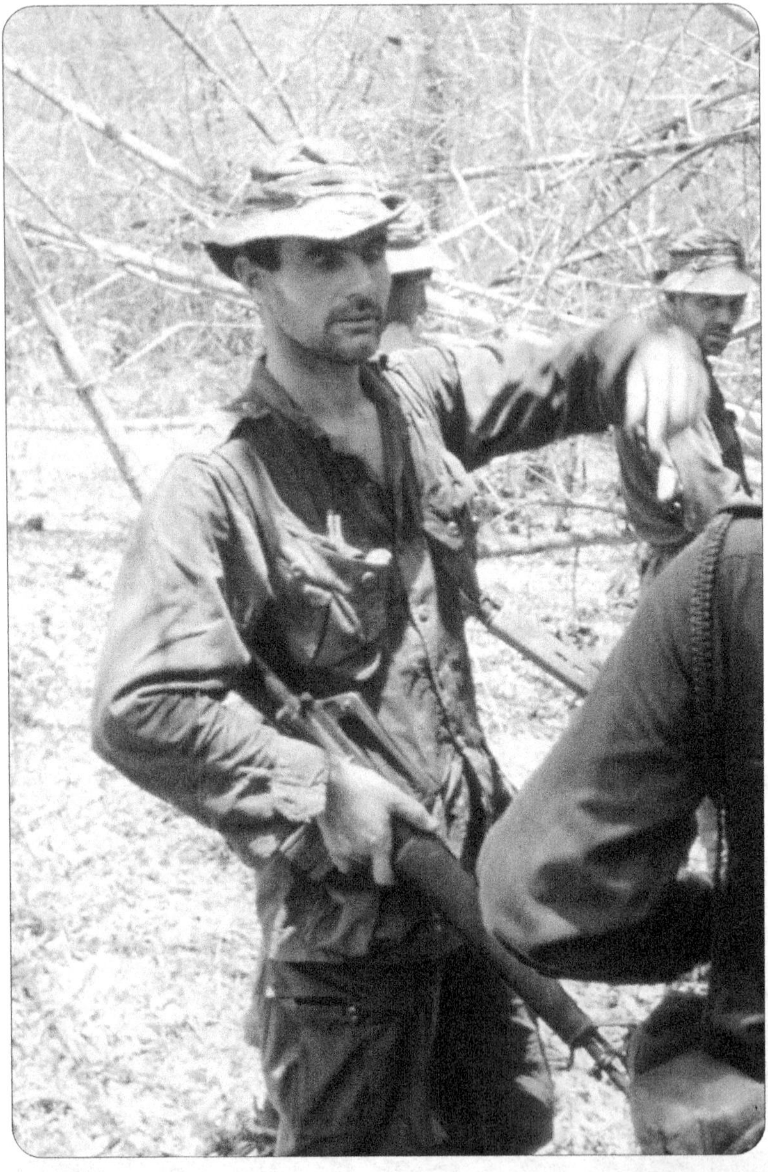

Coburg. An excellent soldier, leader and was largely responsible for our low number of casualties. His men would have followed him anywhere.

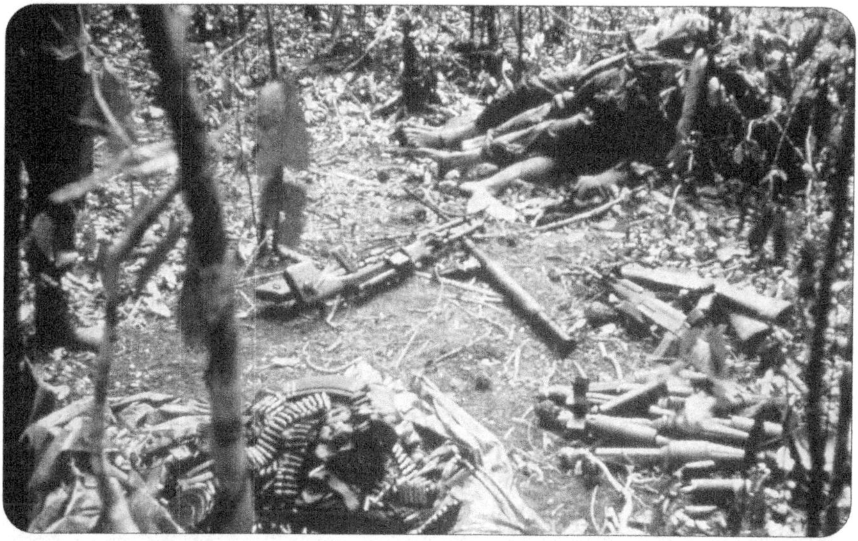

VC dead and captured weapons from the battle on February 7, when V2 company was attacked by a large enemy force. The VC with elements of North Vietnamese regulars engaged the New Zealanders from all sides with heavy automatic and rocket fire. After two hours of intense combat, the VC withdrew with heavy losses. V Company suffered only 10 wounded, 3 serious.

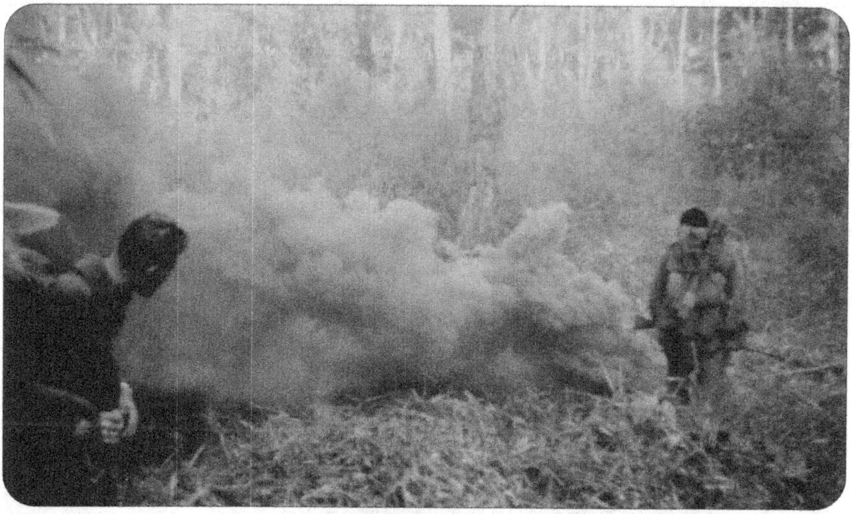

Steve Vautier (left) signalling with smoke grenade to incoming 'dust off' helicopter to find us, to evacuate the wounded and for resupply during Operation Coburg. February 1968.

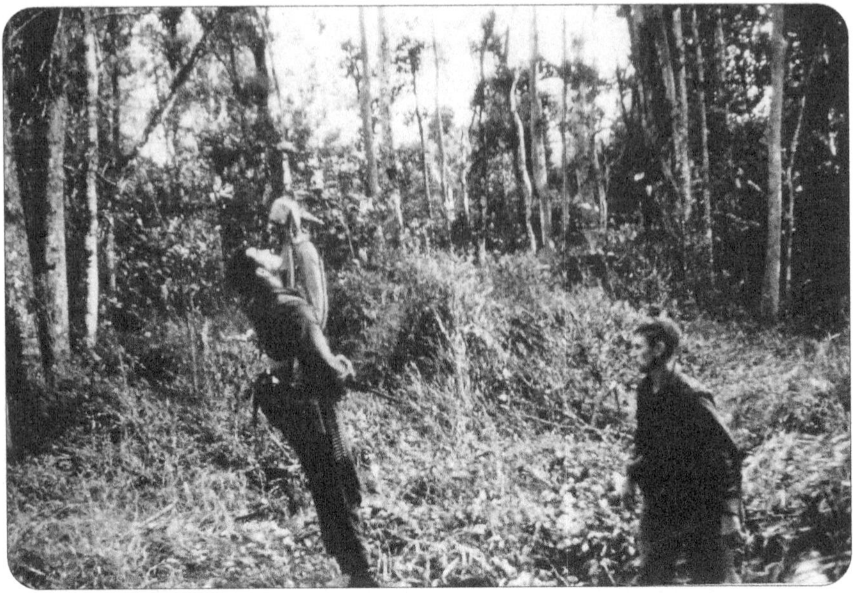

Wounded and sick being air-lifted out by 'dust-off' helicopter during Coburg. Left unknown, right Blue Neame.

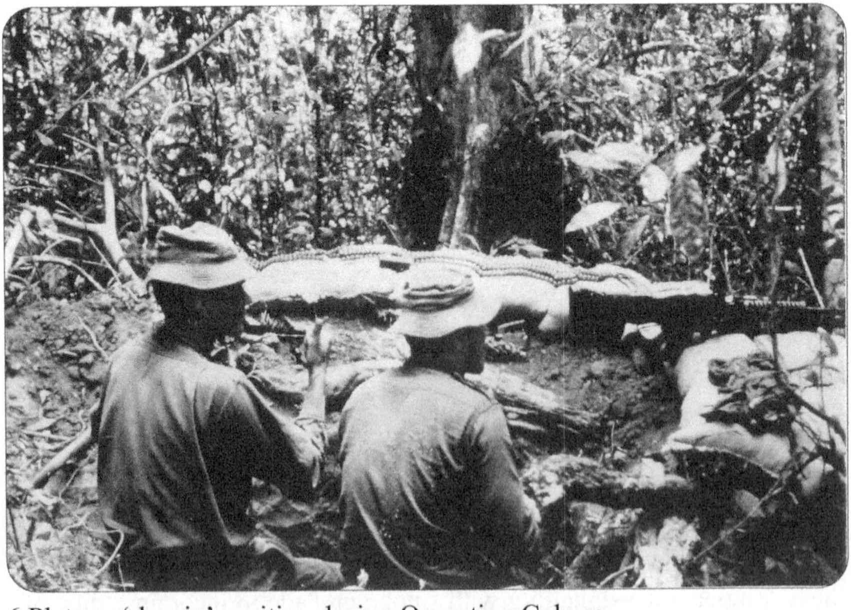

6 Platoon 'dug-in' position during Operation Coburg.

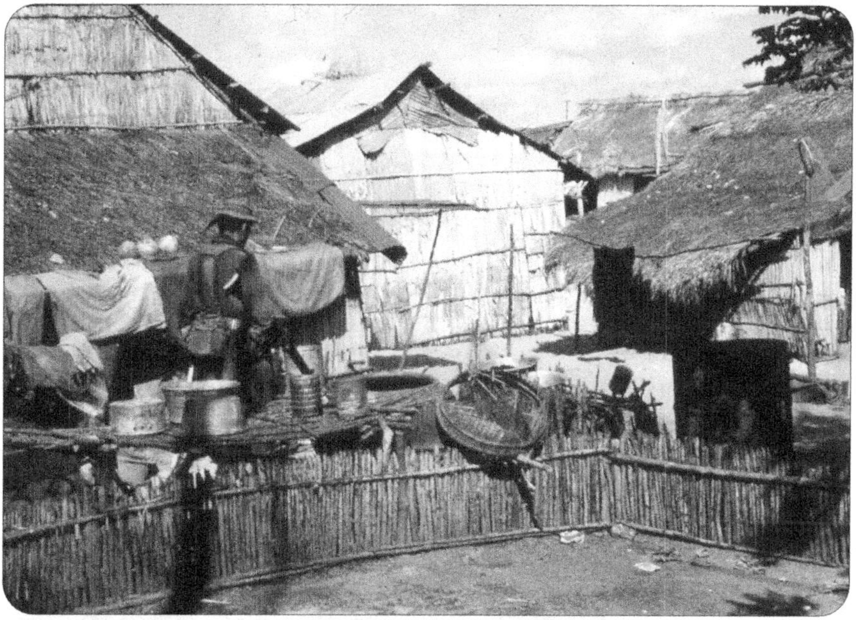

Operation Oakleigh, search and cordon of the village of Hoa Long. February 1968

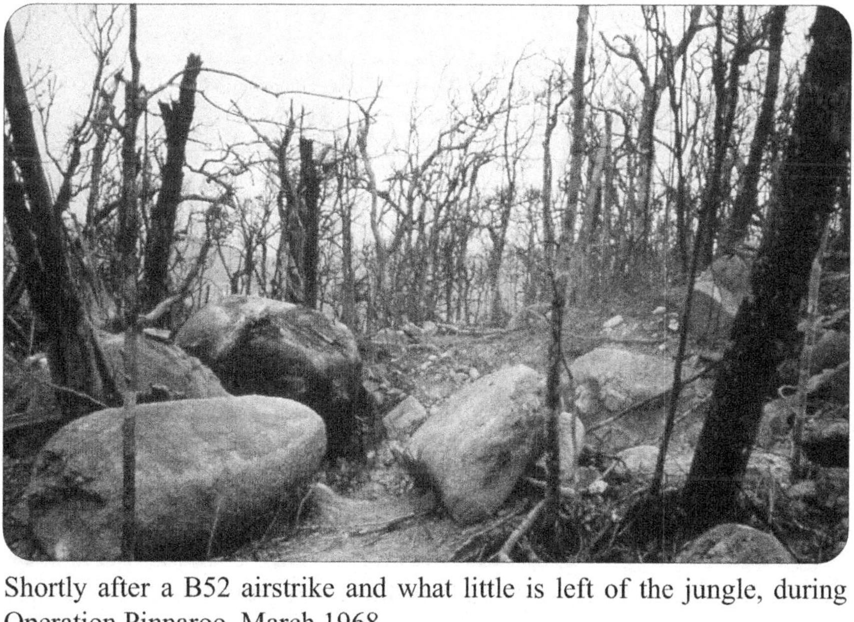

Shortly after a B52 airstrike and what little is left of the jungle, during Operation Pinnaroo. March 1968.

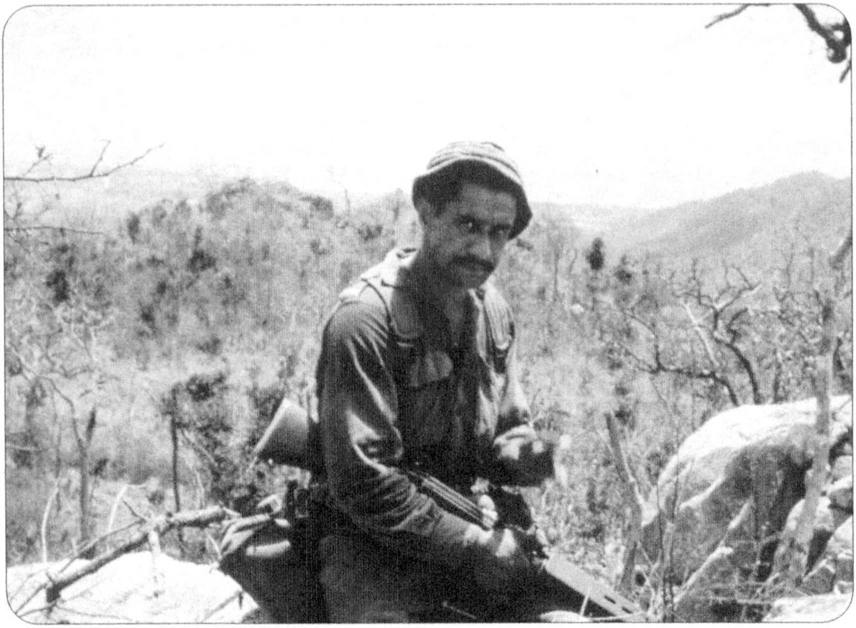

Barney Tautau, one of the best lead scouts in the Company.
March 1968.

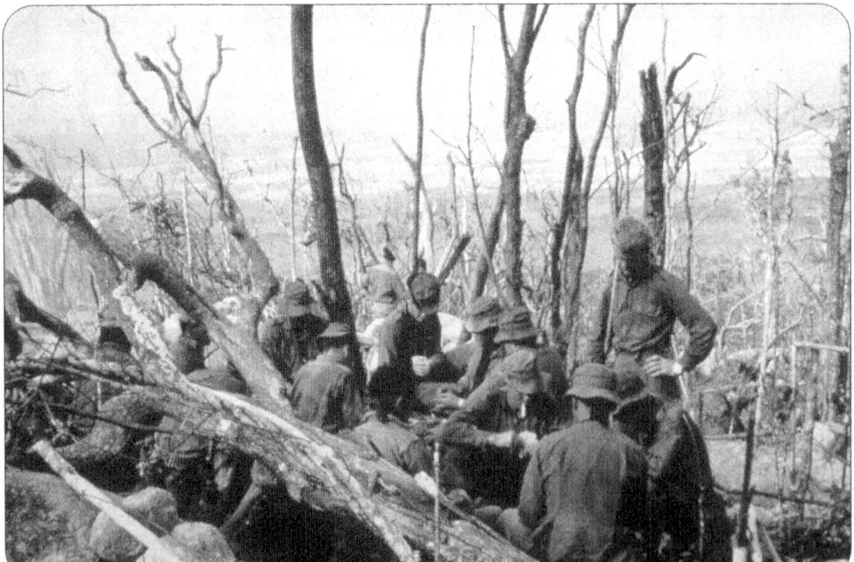

Six Platoon occupying the heights in the Long Hai Hills after massive airstrikes during Pinnaroo.

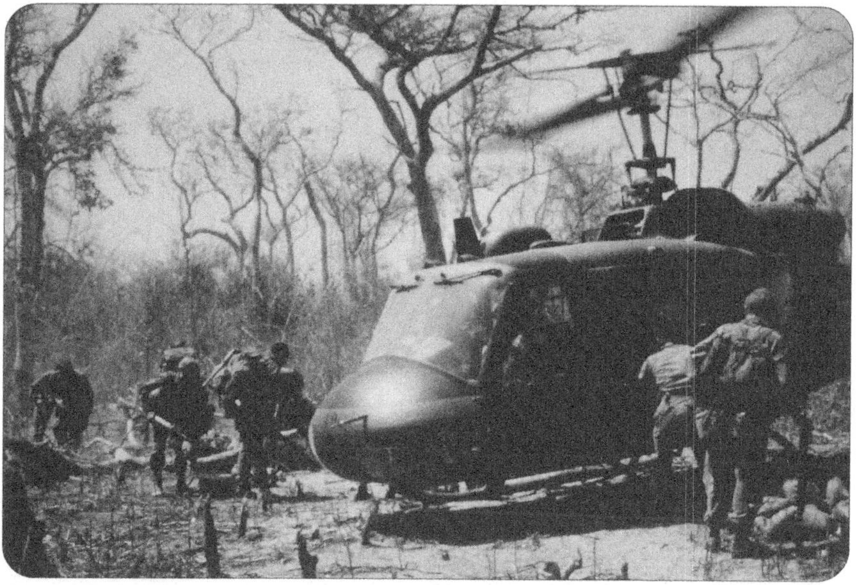

Six Platoon completing Pinnaroo, being picked up by Hueys and returning to Nui Dat.

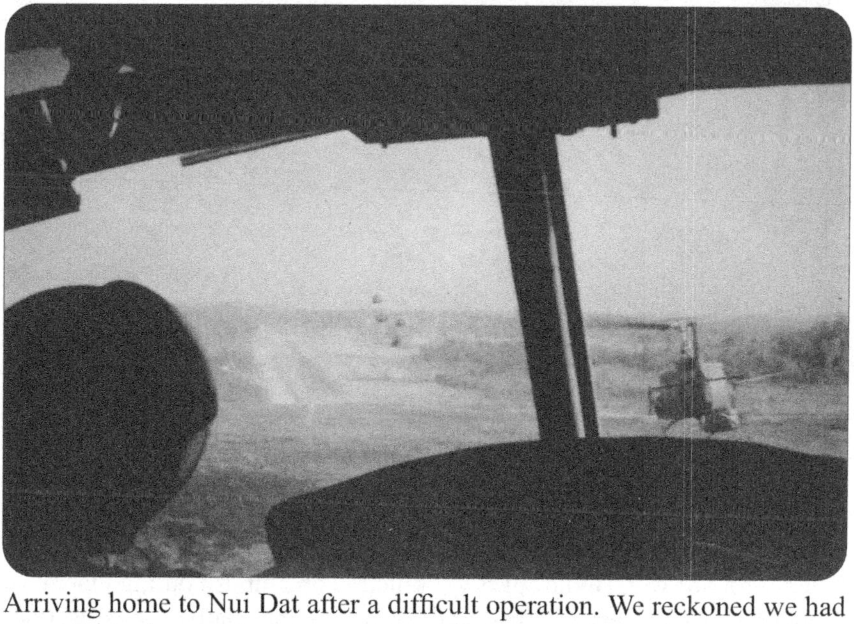

Arriving home to Nui Dat after a difficult operation. We reckoned we had earned ourselves a hot shower and a cold beer. April 1968.

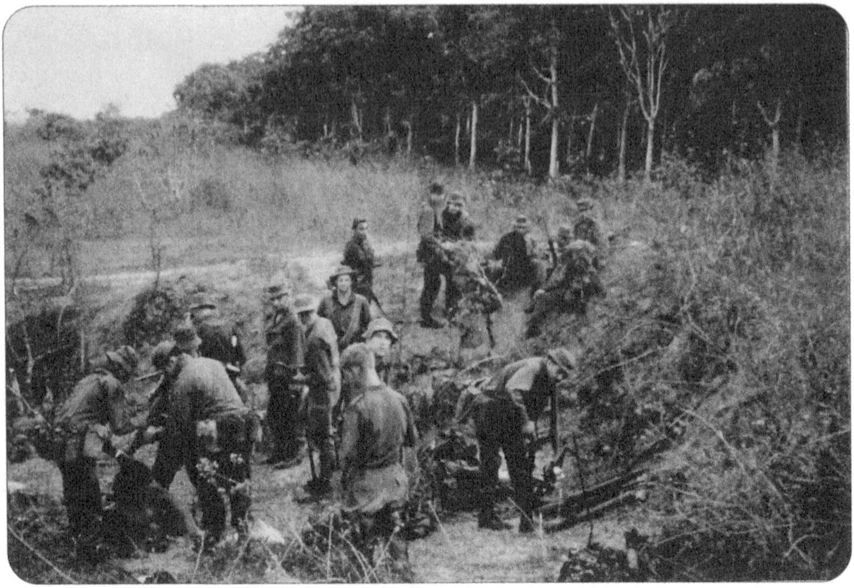

Six Platoon, morning after an ambush that killed 6 VC, April 1968.

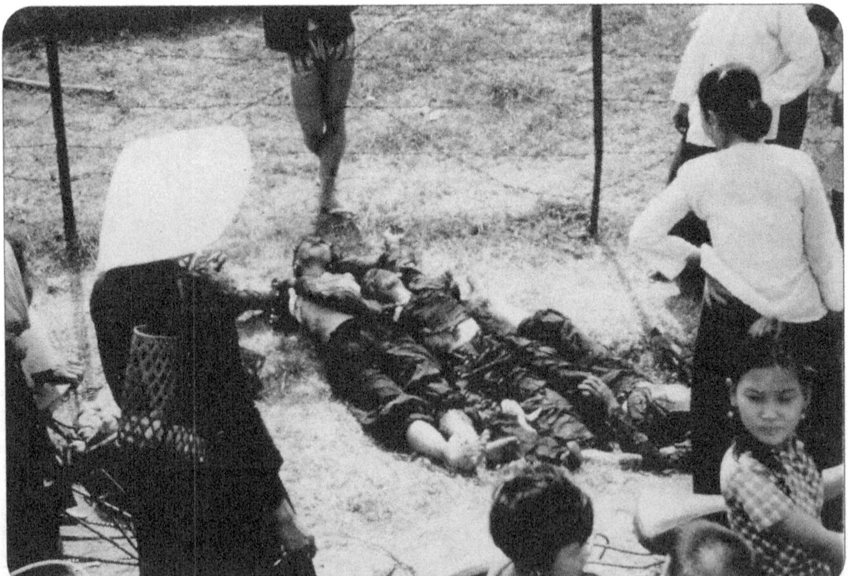

The horrors of war. Bodies of 6 VC killed in an ambush during Operation Cooktown. They were returned to their village for relatives to collect and bury. April 1968

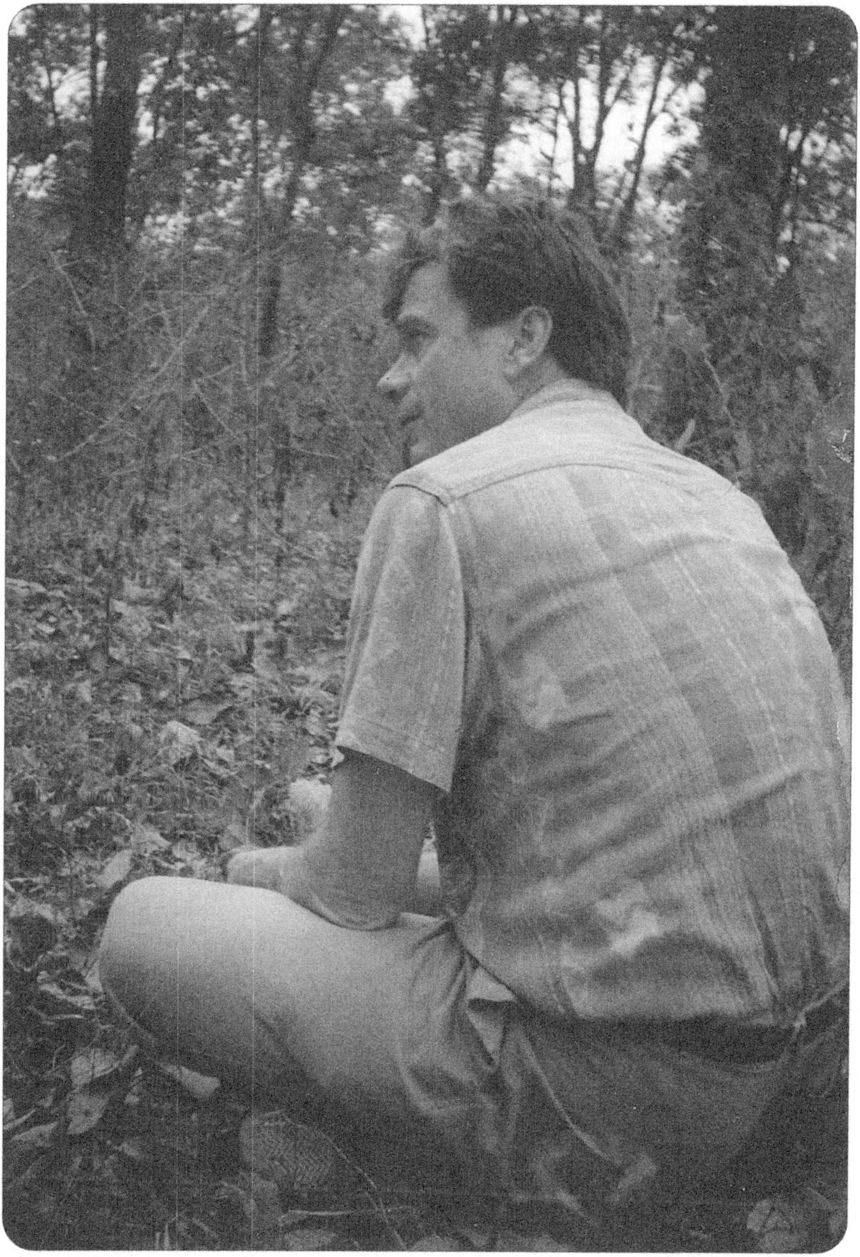

The Author returns to Vietnam 25 years later. His closing ceremony on his wounded warrior status. February 1st, 1993

16

THE VC ARE HUMAN AFTER ALL

The dust-off helicopter lifted off with four dead ARVN and the wounded officer and flew back to their base. We heard later that the officer died of his wounds.

Either we or the ARVN had been in the wrong place to allow such an accident to happen. It was standard procedure that only one friendly unit operated in any area at night. We waited for an hour, giving other ARVN units in the area time to leave and thus avoid further accidental contacts. We then moved to re-join the other half of our platoon, who were concerned, having only heard that there were four dead and one wounded, and so assumed the casualties were us, considering that we had been caught in the ambush. Happily, we could reassure them we were all safe.

The next day was March 7, and we moved towards V Company's position to re-join them. On the way at one rest stop, the attention of the platoon was drawn to our two commanders, as their voices became raised in a heated argument. Hamish Wilson and Sgt. John Whitworth was discussing and then disagreeing on the return route to V Company's position. Eventually, Whitworth stormed away, calling the platoon to their feet for them to follow him. Wilson, with his hands on his hips, determined to assert his authority, shouted after him, his voice very official.

"Come back here, Sergeant Whitworth."

Whitworth kept walking, convinced that he was right. Every one of us looked at each other, trying to decide whom to follow, for a wrong decision could mean mutiny and a court martial. They shoot people for that. A look of indecision flickered over Wilson's face, then his body relaxed, a sign of inner resolve. Each man in the platoon slowly stood up and made his decision. All Whitworth's group followed him down the track, whilst the rest of us stayed with Wilson. Without a further word, we set off to re-join V Company, using an alternative route. Under normal situations, it was standard jungle warfare procedure to never use the same track twice. It was customary for VC units to set ambushes on tracks that allied troops had used, hoping they would return using that track again. Many American units had already become victims of such situations. But these were not normal times.

On our arrival two hours later, there was no time for the two men to settle their differences. After being resupplied, we moved north to RV (rendezvous) with a squadron of APCs that were to carry us on the following day into the next phase of Operation Pinnaroo. Wilson and Whitworth formed an unspoken truce and, though they were very cool and official to each other, they conducted themselves throughout the following operation as true professionals. The outcome of their disagreement was never made known, but Wilson was posted a month later, suggesting that HQ had sided with Whitworth.

Later that afternoon, a B52 bombing strike occurred about five kilometres from our position to the south in the Long Hai hills. Without warning, a line of large spouts of dirt, dust and smoke suddenly erupted fifty metres into the air, to be followed many seconds later by a thunderous boom. It was a very spectacular sight. Such an attack must have been dreadful for the enemy. The aircraft were so high they could barely be seen or heard and gave no warning of the terrible destruction they were about to rain down.

The Long Hai hills, and the peninsula jutting out into the sea, had long been an established base for various VC district and irregular guerrilla units. In addition, units of D445, a Provincial VC mainline battalion, were stationed there to support local VC units in their attacks against the surrounding population centres. The enemy had heavily mined and booby-trapped the entire area and were warned to be extra cautious. 2 and 3 RAR battalions, with APCs and tanks, were to clear the entire area in a search and destroy operation. Pinnaroo, in fact, started on February 27 with the clearing of Long Dien village, and escalated into a full task force operation. Our role was to set up ambushes, help clear areas of VC camps and eventually prevent enemy units from retreating. This would happen as 2 RAR and support units began a sweep towards our dug-in positions. It was a similar plan to Operation Duntroon months earlier and was hoped that it would meet with the same success.

After being dropped off by the APCs, we moved into the foothills. Within an hour of being dropped off, the 'thumbs down' signal came back from our lead scout. Without orders, we fell into an impromptu 'spread out' and ambush position, ready to strike. It impressed me at our professionalism that came from the practise of so many contacts over the last few months.

Within a minute, a bullock cart with an old Vietnamese gentleman and a young child about eight years old appeared on the track coming towards us. The oxen pulling the cart, with its large bell clanging from under its neck, slowly approached, unaware of thirty-six men ready to blow them away.

'Surely the boss will not order us to spring the ambush, or was he? These people are obviously civilians,' I thought with a rising concern as they approached. Just then, Hamish Wilson stepped onto the track with his hand raised and ordered the Vietnamese to go back, for they were in a restricted area. I felt relieved.

For the next week, the Long Hai hills took a dreadful pounding from artillery fire and massive airstrikes by an assortment of aircraft, including more B52 bombers. Every day, we could hear combat as elements of our clearing force engaged pockets of VC scattered throughout the hills as they approached us.

It was extremely hot moving through many areas, for the jungle had been stripped of most of its foliage during the bombardments and offered little shade from the sun. As warned, mines were a problem, but we had Australian engineers with us, acting as minefield clearing teams, and using mine-detectors. Their efforts were invaluable and probably saved us from many injuries and loss of life judging from the many mines and booby-traps that they found in our path.

On the 11th, we set up an all-day ambush, and I made sure that I found a position in the shade under some scattered bush. After lying there for an hour, the sun moved, and my shade disappeared. Unable to move, the sweat poured off me and the heat made me drowsy. It was hard to stay awake, but I knew the importance of doing so while in an ambush position. Charlie could appear without warning. Being sleep deprived from evening sentry duty every night, the heat of the day found me slowly drifting in and out of dozing.

Suddenly I was instantly awake as I felt Blue's hand firmly touching my leg, warning me of danger. I did not remember him being that close to me. I could not see any enemy to my immediate front. Slowly, not to make a sudden move that would give my position away to an approaching enemy, I turned my head to look at him, to see where he was looking. But he was nowhere in sight. Alarmed, I carefully looked down to see who was touching me, and to my horror saw that a large brown snake had crawled onto my leg. It appeared to be about two metres long, with black stripes on its body, and probably had mistaken me for a log. I froze, and ever so slowly, I lowered my face into the red dust and waited. I desperately tried to control my emotions, knowing that all creatures react to fear. My body became saturated with sweat as I wrestled with my mind going into overdrive with craziness. My machete attached to my webbing was out of reach by the way I was lying and to manoeuvre myself in reaching it would cause too much movement, alerting the creature to possibly attack.

Then the snake crawled slowly up my leg and onto my buttocks. I dared not breathe. Its weight, pressing down on my body, was surprisingly heavy. It seemed to stay there forever, motionless. The thought of it suddenly burying its fangs into my thigh kept screaming through my mind. Time passed infinitely slowly, and I was sure that the reptile could hear the beating of my heart. I gently lifted my head, glanced at my watch, and lowered it again, ever so slowly. I would give it 15 minutes and then quietly call for help was the only strategy I could think of.

After about 10 minutes, it started moving again, and it slithered into the small of my back. Then I felt its weight lighten as it began leaving my body. As soon as it was not touching any other part of me, slowly I turned my head and saw it moving away. Quickly I rolled in the opposite direction, and my sudden movement caused the snake to rear up in fright, ready to strike, but it saw I was out of striking range and quickly slithered away.

"Who's making that noise?" I heard Paddy Perawiti hiss.

"F_ck your noise. I nearly got eaten by a bloody ten-ton snake." I hissed back.

"Settle down, you blokes," came Steve Vautier's soothing but authoritative voice. An hour later, we were relieved from the ambush site. I had seen many snakes, particularly in Malaysia, during our jungle warfare training. Because we moved so slowly, we often came across and remarkably close to many jungle animals. But that was the closest and the most terrifying encounter with any such creature.

Later that day, looking down into the valley far below, we spotted a lone bullock cart moving along a dirt track leading into our restricted area. It was probably a local farmer out to get some firewood, but it could be a

VC on some surveillance mission. Hamish Wilson called in mortar fire to frighten the supposed farmer into moving back to the safety of the road. The first shell fell about 200 metres away to his right, and he stopped, as if deciding whether or not to go on. Then three more shells landed in front of him, much closer, causing him to turn his cart around and bolt back along the track at intense speed. Ben Hur and his chariot had nothing on that speeding Vietnamese and his 'Grand Prix' winning bullock! The sight of the swiftly retreating peasant was so comical that we all doubled up with laughter. Eventually, the poor guy reached the road and was lost in a cloud of dust, never to be seen again.

Two Australian engineers blew down some trees with high explosives to help clear a chopper landing zone. Directly afterwards, the strong acrid smell of cordite, the aftermath of detonating high explosives, hung in the air, and I wanted to throw up. It struck me that it was the same smell that lingered after every battle. Such a smell had become associated with death, fear, and terribly mutilated bodies.

On the 17th, we joined up with Five Platoon and, at midday, began moving higher into the Long Hai hills. A massive B52 bombing strike was made on the top of the hill where our objective was. The sky was blotted out by a heavy dust cloud and, a minute later, dust and particles came raining down on us, covering our sweat-sodden shirts and faces. American jet fighter bombers followed this, strafing with cannon fire and dropping napalm bombs on VC positions. Their cannons sounded like heavy furniture being dragged along a wooden floor. Their napalm, when it exploded, dealt an instant and hideous death to anyone caught in it. The horror of such an end refreshed my already nightly nightmares during my restless sleep.

It was just before dark when we arrived at the top. There was no sign of any VC or anything else. Barely a tree remained standing and huge rocks had been ripped from the earth in the wake of the heavy bombardments. We were all exhausted, short of water, and very dirty from the climb. Most of us collapsed where we were, too tired to dig shell scrapes, and just lay on the bare ground and quickly went to sleep, interrupted only by two hours of sentry duty.

By the next morning, most of us had completely run out of water, and with no shade, the conditions were intolerable. Throughout the day I sucked on fruit drops, candy from our Australian supplied ration packs to fend off the pangs of thirst. We had not shaved or showered since the 27th of the previous month, three weeks earlier. The shortage of water in the last week meant that we couldn't even wash our hands and faces, and

I feared my dysentery might return. By now, we were used to the smell of each other, but our skins itched from the weeks of accumulated sweat and grime. Tempers were raw and arguments would flare up for the most trivial reasons. Despite the obvious hardships, it was the constant exposure to combat, or the threat of it, that played heavily on even the strongest amongst us. No one was immune.

Late that afternoon, a Huey came in with the mail and a resupply of water – the most delicious I had ever tasted. A letter arrived from my mother and another from my brother, Warwick. It was good to hear from them. Mail from home always lifted morale.

Throughout the day, the sounds of battle raged in different locations throughout the Long Hai hills, as the Australians and New Zealand's W Company mopped up pockets of the enemy. The battle sounds were so constant that we largely ignored them. We were ever ready for the retreating VC units to stumble into our well-dug-in and ambush positions.

The monotony between duties and frayed nerves was relieved by two unofficial unit clowns. Most Australian and Kiwi platoons had one, but we were blessed with two. Colin Burgering, and Danny McPhail, our second platoon radio operator. Danny would come out with the most extraordinary scientific statements about the most mundane things. He would make some hilarious points, while all the time keeping a profoundly serious face expression, which made him even funnier. "I don't need food. I'm solar-powered," was his only comment about the lack of shade.

I could enjoy Colin's company more often, as we were in the same section. He had an endless supply of jokes, and being English, his accent made his jokes even funnier.

On one of our patrols, we came across several ancient Vietnamese temples that must have been over a thousand years old. They were hidden in deep patches of jungle and were covered in dense undergrowth and strangled by the roots of old trees. Unfortunately, they had been partly destroyed from the B52 strike, and we would have missed them, except that much of the overgrown vegetation had been blown away by the blasts. I wanted to examine them more closely, as no doubt this was an important archaeological find. Regrettably, there was no time to do so, and the patrol continued.

No enemy ventured in our direction during this time. Except one night, while I was alone on sentry duty. The boss wanted to rest the guys as much as possible by only putting one sentry on at a time, instead of the usual two.

Suddenly, I heard the animated voices of two VC less than 20 metres from where I was sitting. Judging from the loudness of their voices, they did not know we were here. Not seeing them in the darkness, I pulled a hand grenade from my webbing in readiness to pull the pin and toss it in their direction, knowing it will probably kill them both. Then, I could hear a woman's as well as a man's voice and they were having an argument, which sounded like a lover's quarrel. My heart went out to them, and I placed my grenade back on my webbing. I wanted to warn them to leave before they woke up the rest of the platoon, who would probably be less understanding. I thought of making a noise to frighten them off, but that could put my own life in danger.

I smiled as she seemed to accuse him of something as he gently tried to reason with her. Being in rapid Vietnamese and not understanding a word, but it was clear to what they were saying to each other. It made me want to laugh out loud at this very human interaction.

Just then, a sound from one of our guys stirring in his sleep alerted them and they silently disappeared into the night. Feeling relieved that they were now safe, I suddenly noticed a strange idea that the VC were actual people instead of just being 'Charlie,' the enemy to kill! I often wondered if they survived the war and if they ever reached a resolution over their squabble. I hope so on both counts.

Being unsure if I broke any military codes, and I never enquired. This was a restricted area, meaning that any Vietnamese in this area would be VC and standing orders were to attack them at every opportunity. But, in my heart, it felt the right thing.

17

WINNERS AND LOSERS

Early on the morning of 21st March, I and one other were flown back by Huey to Nui Dat, where we enjoyed a twenty-four-hour leave and the luxury of my first shower, a beer and a comfortable bed for nearly a month. As the company was returning to Nui Dat in two days, we could stay on and took the opportunity to thoroughly clean all my equipment and my two weapons, but my mind was on other things. It seemed that back at base, I could relax from being so mindful and attentive while on patrol. This was to have dire consequences.

During this time, I had a check-up with the Doctor about the state of my dysentery, which seemed stable for now. He decided I can remain on active duty, because of the shortage of personnel, but to report to him the moment the symptoms re-appeared. That might be difficult if I am out in the field on an operation. He shrugged as if that was a minor matter, and I dropped the issue. Even though I was being plagued at night with regular nightmares, I still wanted to complete the tour of duty. My dreams at night were the worst part of this overall experience. I was becoming hardened to the actual combat and there was a small part of me that 'got off' from the adrenalin rush with each contact. 'You must be one sick bastard to gather even the slightest pleasure from all this craziness,' I thought to myself.

I was tempted to ask the Doctor about the weird experience of everything slowing down in the middle of a firefight that had now happened twice. This was an older and more experienced Doctor than the last one. But decided against it in case he reported it, had me certified as unfit for combat and sent home. I think I know how to control it now, and if I can stay reasonably sane for the rest of my tour, I can get psychological help when I get back to New Zealand, was my thought.

On the 25th and 26th V company took part in Operation Ashgrove Tram, another cordon and search of the village of Xa Long Hai, situated at the foot of the Long Hai hills and on the coast. High command believed that the VC had been driven from the Long Hai hills during the last operation and may have sought refuge in this small and isolated fishing village.

As we drove out of Nui Dat in trucks, we were ordered as usual to cock our weapons, for readiness to fire. As I cocked my M16 rifle, a round ejected out of the breach, showing that it was already loaded. Hamish Wilson saw this.

"Was your weapon already cocked inside Nui Dat, Sisson?" he demanded, knowing that Standing Orders said as a safety precaution, that no weapons were to be cocked within Nui Dat.

"No sir," I lied. "I cocked it just before."

I turned away in horror, realising that I had been carrying a fully loaded weapon in Nui Dat for five days. My neglect was made worse because I hadn't even put the safety catch on. How could this have happened?

In a moment of distraction or daydreaming, while cleaning the M16, I had cocked it with the magazine in, and a round had automatically been loaded into the breach. With this weapon, you can't put the safety catch on unless it is cocked, and I didn't think to check this. Such a lethal moment to depart from my usual mindfulness, and probably some influence from the stress of PTSD.

On this current operation we were part of the search team, but it was a relatively quiet affair with only nine VC suspects being detained from the screening process. Since Tet and Operation Pinnaroo, the Communists in Phuoc Tuy Province, as with most of the country, had been well and truly defeated, as VC activity had dropped dramatically.

Back in Nui Dat, John Linley had his 21st birthday, an occasion for a hilarious night of letting off steam. Blue got arrested for striking an officer while drunk and was sentenced to twenty-one days in the 'lockup. Several of us had to escort him and another prisoner from W Company to Vung Tau prison. The road from Nui Dat to Vung Tau, once regarded as dangerous from VC ambush, was now relatively quiet. Nevertheless, our two Land Rovers travelled very fast to lessen the danger from mines and snipers. At the prison, I got angry when I saw how the Australian Military police treated Blue as they escorted him away. If only they had known how amazing he was in every firefight, I think they would have shown him more respect.

We stopped for a few beers while in Vung Tau, and I expressed my anger over Blue's treatment. Then we drove back to Nui Dat. On the way, our second vehicle, driven by Tom Whitaker, got held up behind a local civilian car whose driver would not let him pass. After repeated horn blowing and attempts to pass, and all the time falling dangerously further behind our vehicle, Tom stuck his rifle out of the window and put a shot over the car in front. This action instantly had the desired effect of forcing the offending driver to pull over, so that Tom could pass and catch up with us.

"A good trick against painfully slow drivers. I must remember that when I get home," someone in our vehicle commented drily.

Life in Nui Dat settled down to cleaning equipment, filling sandbags to reinforce protection around our tents and other uninteresting chores.

Lining up for meals at the mess tent (yummy fresh food after ration field packs for so long) it was common for the guys to play word games and quick reflex games, to fill in time whilst waiting. In one reflex game, a player had to try to hit his opponent's hand as he quickly withdrew it the split second, he saw his opponent move to strike his hand. One lunchtime line-up, I was playing with one guy, Bill, from four platoon. He was a big man, and I was too fast for him to strike my hand as I withdrew it. Each time he tried to hit it, his frustration caused his arm movements to become wilder with each attempt, until one accidentally connected with my jaw and knocked me clean out. I woke up a few seconds later, on the ground with Bill standing over me, with a worried look on his face. The rest of the guys waiting in line were laughing. As I stood up shakily, someone joked.

"Hey Sas, you don't want to play that with Bill, because if he can't win, he just knocks your bloody head off." This caused further laughter, and I joined in, as I sheepishly rubbed my jaw.

The days ran into each other, with little breaking the monotony. On April the 1st, Sgt Major Hayward, Andy, Graham, three Australian mortar crew and I drove outside the wire and blew up sixty old mortar shells, numerous grenades and an assortment of unserviceable mines, ammunition, and claymores. Having been trained in demolition during my time with the SAS, this was good practice for my skills. We all enjoyed the big bang.

Hamish Wilson was posted and replaced by Lt. Mountfort. I always thought that Wilson went 'too much by the book' and lacked flexibility with his men regarding discipline and day-to-day running of the platoon. But his leadership and courage during the heaviest of the fighting proved to me he was a fine soldier and officer. I found, somewhat to my surprise, that I later missed him. Mountfort was much more relaxed and easier to get on with, in everyday affairs, but his leadership skills were never tested in battle as Wilson's were. Yet, there was nothing about him that caused us to doubt him. The quality of leadership in V company at all levels was generally very high.

That night, while playing cards in our tent, Four platoon's M60 machine gun suddenly opened fire from its sentry position close to the wire. "Stand to, Charlie's on the wire." All lights were turned out as we grabbed our weapons and sprinted to our forward trenches. Several VC had been seen probing our defences, a sharp reminder that we were still in a war and there were still Viet Cong out there. No enemy casualties were found and the order to stand down came an hour later.

"You know," Duggan said as we walked back to our tents,

"I bet those Charlie bastards knew I had the winning hand right at that point."

"Yeah, I paid them to come in at that exact moment," someone answered.

On April 3, we moved out in trucks on Operation Cooktown Orchid. The object of this operation was to clear all remaining VC from the jungle area immediately surrounding the Long Hai hills. The mission was to set up a series of ambushes further to the north, intercept retreating or VC reinforcements to the main operational area.

Despite the VC probing our wire defences in Nui Dat, we didn't expect to see anything, still believing that the war is all but over. For the next two days, we split the platoon as previously, so that the Platoon could cover two ambush sites per night. On the night of the 5th, we found an old abandoned and empty water reservoir, about 30 metres long by 15 metres wide, with earth banks about two metres high. Several tracks converged on this site, making it ideal for an ambush site.

Just before midnight, I was on the north-eastern corner as a sentry with the M60 machine gun, when I heard the movement of a large number of VC approaching through the abandoned rubber plantation to my front. I pulled the communication cord connecting each sentry position, alerting Colin Burgering on the southeast corner, and Toy (David) Rawiri on the west side. The response tug was returned from Toy's position, but not from Colin's. I pulled his again a little stronger only to hear a loud clunk sound from Colin's position. When first setting up the ambush, he had tied his end of the communication cord to the radio aerial. When he received my alarm signal, he forgot to reply with the customary response tug and quickly went to wake up his section. My second stronger tug on the cord pulled the radio set over with a resounding 'clunk'. He quickly returned and now pulled the response tug. Meantime, 'Toy' was waking up his squad, as I was mine, but I feared that our position might be already compromised with the sound of the falling wireless set. I listened and at the time of the radio falling over, the enemy had stopped, alerted by the sound. After a pause of about 30 seconds they began moving again, as I could once more hear many pairs of feet approaching our position.

I could feel the excitement as adrenalin pumped through my veins. Dick Dargaville silently took over his M60 from me and I moved with my M79 grenade launcher to a better firing position along to the left side of the reservoir bank.

Sgt. Whitworth quietly arrived beside me, whispering.

"How many are there, Sas?"

"It sounds like at least a platoon, but could be a company," I softly whispered back.

"Shit. That is a serious problem, because they could overrun us here if we hit them."

Kneeling on the ground next to him, I knew what he was thinking, as it echoed my own thoughts.

'Small VC squads of 8 or less run from all contacts. But a platoon size or bigger, if hit by a smaller force and at such a close quarter, are likely to immediately attack and over-run us.' I too whispered, "Shit."

By now, the sound of enemy movement was all around us, with some directly on the other side of the bank, two metres away.

From the corner of my eye, I suddenly saw a VC climb onto the top of the wall and was looking down on the 16 of us. Before he could cry out a warning to his comrades, one of our guys fired off a cluster of claymores. They shattered the night stillness with a deafening explosion. Sparks, dust, and wetness of what must have been nightly moisture from the top of the reservoir bank from the erupting claymores covered us. The VC disappeared as the blast blew him to pieces and everyone opened fire. The decision to hit them or not was out of our hands and the dice had been cast.

Ratima, with his M79, and I with mine, started peppering the surrounding area with grenades. After a minute, I moved to another position for a better field of fire. I noticed that my face and hands were wet and sticky. Several minutes later, when there was no further enemy movement, we stopped firing. Whitworth's voice called out.

"Sisson, come over here, quick."

I sprinted to his side.

"Come with me." I followed him to the northern end of the reservoir, where moaning sounds twenty metres away could be heard near the rubber plantation.

"Silence, the bastard, will you," he commanded. As I adjusted my sights in the moonlight, in preparation to fire towards several heaps on the ground where the moans were coming from, we heard someone uttering a gurgling noise on the other side of the bank. We both climbed the mound, and as I fired a grenade towards the rubber trees, John Whitworth emptied his magazine into a wounded VC lying two metres out from our position.

Realising that I only had 3 M79 grenades left, and I may still need them if the VC returned, which they had done in the past after an initial firefight, especially if they are a large force. Sighting my M16 rifle at a moaning and grotesquely twitching form on the ground, I fired, seeing my shots strike with a shudder effect and then moved on to each body. After 20 shots, there was no movement or sound from any of them.

There was no feeling inside of me. I had made them just a 'thing' to emotionally survive and do my job. I could not afford to remember the recent event of the two delightful quarrelling VC lovers.

With all enemy silenced, Whitworth ordered five men to do a sweep of the immediate surrounding area, with the rest of us covering them.

I sat there watching our search team inspect each body as they got to it and gather their weapons. I considered that perhaps why they retreated, rather than overrun us was because of our claymores, two machine guns, two M79 grenade launchers and 12 small arms fire, so sudden and all at once probably gave the enemy the impression that we were a bigger force than we were.

The pungent and familiar stench of cordite and death hung in the air. I had no feelings for or against those dead enemy soldiers. We had won, and they had lost, having paid the ultimate price. Just another contact. Again, luck was on our side. Had the situation been even slightly different, it could very well have been our bodies lying there being searched.

Joe Hoani caught my attention, being part of the inspection team, and found a VC who seemed to be still alive, but in the dark, he wasn't sure. Joe picked up the VC's Thompson sub-machine gun, aimed at the slightly twitching form, and fired until the magazine was empty.

This reflected another thought of how uncompromising the Vietnam war had been. Very few prisoners had been taken, and only those who had not been badly wounded had interrogation value. This sparked the moral question to resurface. Are we fighting an honourable war? Is any war honourable? Perhaps the Second World War against the Nazi holocaust, maybe? With horror, I realised we had become so emotionally wounded that we could now kill so effortlessly. I tried to justify myself with the thought that to kill a man who was still alive, but terribly mutilated from the effects of modern gunshot wounds was an act of compassion. Especially from claymore mines that literally stripped every thread of flesh from a man's body. Death was a merciful release from such suffering.

Perhaps it would be better if the destruction and suffering caused by war were so terrible, no prisoners, total genocide become the norm, that eventually everyone would wake up to its insanity. Perhaps this would end war forever? I am sure I am not the first person to have had such a thought and yet, war has been raging almost non-stop for 20,000 years and we haven't woken up. Besides, there would be people who would use such total war as a justification that their side was 'right,' and the other side was in the wrong and needed punishment. People would always find a justification to hold on to their beliefs at all costs. Perhaps this is where the answer lies. What if everyone stopped believing in a cause that they will kill for? Would people go to war believing in nothing?

Such questioning and pacifist thinking was putting me in an impossible position. I closed the lid on such thoughts, at least until I leave Vietnam.

Six bodies were found. Several small fires were burning, set off by the blasts from the claymores and M79 grenades. Half of the squad stood to on sentry duty for the rest of the night in case the VC returned. The next morning, I was greeted with the stench of something unfamiliar and unpleasant. As I sat up and glanced down my front, I realised with revulsion that I was splattered with blood, bits of human skin, fragments of bone, and brains were stuck to my shirt, face, and hands. The VC opposite the bank where I had been standing when the claymores were fired had been blown to pieces like a watermelon by the claymore blast right next to him, and I had been showered with parts of his anatomy. Feeling nauseated, I quickly emptied my water bottle over my head and hands and, with my bayonet, scraped the fragments off my shirt.

We did another sweep and inspected the dead more thoroughly for documents and equipment. Some were wearing civilian clothes; others were partly in combat dress. Only one was dressed in the full black VC uniform. There was several blood-smeared drag-marks, showing that we inflicted more casualties on them. Trying not to vomit, I sat silently on the ground, listening to the guys discuss the matter. One looked at me.

"Hey Sas, are you collecting body parts?" The others laughed.

"Every time I turn around you are covered in splattered blood and this time parts of a Charlie,"

"Well, you know Sas," Colin Burgering chipped in. "He throws himself into his work, literally."

I enjoyed the good-natured mockery but could only manage a weak smile, trying not to vomit. They sensed I was in some emotional pain and sensitively backed off, carrying on with their conversation.

"It seems like Charlie had been coming from the direction of Hoa Long."

"Yeah, and they were probably coming to hit our platoon harbour a kilometre away," Mitch (Mitchell) suggested.

"No, I think they were heading for the Long Hai hills, with all this food they were carrying," IB (Paterson) replied.

"Bloody close to Nui Dat, wouldn't you say?"

"Yeah, it's only about 3 ks from here."

Mitch took a few moments to digest this.

"Shit, maybe Charlie isn't finished, after all."

18

COUNTDOWN TO GOING HOME

Early the next morning, the rest of six platoon arrived at our position and later we moved back to our all-day platoon harbour.

I was feeling physically better, but my mood was fragile. I really am over this whole damn Vietnam experience. 'Just want to go home,' was my only thought. Graham Peddie interrupted my thoughts, arriving beside my shell scrape.

"Did you hear about those VC we killed the other night, Sas?"

"What about them?"

"They were local guerrillas from Hoa Long. One of them was only 15 years old. Blokes from Company HQ took the bodies into Hoa Long and dumped them in the middle of the town for their relatives to bury. I reckon they were also put there as an example to the other locals."

"The poor buggers, the relatives that is." I shuddered at the thought of finding a member of my own family in this way.

"Do you know, Sas, that it's now just over a month before our tour is up?" Graham said with a gleam in his eye.

"You're damn well right," I replied. "I wish we were going home to New Zealand instead of back to Malaysia. Anyway, I can't wait to get back down to Singapore and get rotten."

"Drunk? That's not all I'll be getting."

"Ya randy bugger, no country's going to be safe when they let you out of here. Besides, aren't you going straight home because of your tour to Borneo last year?"

"You bet your bloody sweet life, mate. A few days in Malaysia, and New Zealand, look out." Graham gleefully announced.

Suddenly, life became precious.

"You know, Graham. When I got here five months ago, I would have gladly laid down my life for God, Queen, and Country. I don't think I'm that enthusiastic anymore."

He looked at me for a few seconds, then with a smile got up to move back to his position, saying.

"That would have to be the biggest bloody understatement of the century. See ya 'round."

We spent the next few days patrolling and setting up ambushes each night. But few had any enthusiasm in the war. We all just wanted to go home.

One day while patrolling, I stooped down and picked up one of the propaganda leaflets that littered the countryside. They were distributed both by the VC and the South Vietnamese government. This one had been put out by the North Vietnamese Army, and I hadn't seen this one before. It was written in both Vietnamese and English. With a crudely drawn illustration, showing captive American soldiers with tears streaming down their faces, being escorted away by victorious NVA troops, and read:

'The Imperialist Americans and their lackeys (all the Allied countries were mentioned by name) 'in their futile attempt to prop up the corrupt, illegal government in the South, will be soon defeated.' As I read, a Sioux helicopter with South Vietnamese markings flew overhead, and again, as on every other day, voiced through loudspeakers its propaganda against the Communists. 'Who were these Vietnamese villagers to believe? I don't think the Vietnamese people really care who rules them, so long as the killing and mass destruction is brought to an end.'

Our increasing lack of interest in the war nearly resulted in disaster a few nights later. In the early hours of the morning of April 9, three of us were manning the ambush put in the night before. It was just on 5 a.m. when Colin Burgering leaned over to where I lay.

"Get some sleep, Sas. You, too, Graham. There's no bugger around. I'll keep watch."

"Sounds good to me," I whispered back.

"Yeah, me too." Graham echoed. Both of us rolled over and were fast asleep within a minute. Half an hour later, Colin quietly began to pack up his gear in readiness for the move out at 6.00 am. At that moment, a lone VC walked into the 'killing ground' of the ambush and froze when he heard Colin's movements. Colin saw the VC only five metres away, looking in his direction, but not seeing him. The VC, with his AK47 levelled in our direction, was peering into the darkness straight at Colin, obviously unsure whether he had heard something. Colin dared not move or breathe. To have reached for his rifle, or for the switch of the claymores, would have cost us our lives. Having satisfied himself that his imagination had been playing tricks on him, the VC walked on down the track and out of the ambush site.

I felt Colin's hand on my shoulder and was instantly awake. Slowly and quietly, I rolled over and gripped my rifle. Graham was also alerted. A minute later, a dog trotted into the ambush and began growling and barking at us. We heard a low whistle from the VC down the track, and the dog ran off. We looked at each other embarrassingly. Had we all been awake, the ambush would have been successful, so we kept quiet about this misadventure when we later returned to our platoon harbour.

The next day, news came through that there had been a major disaster in New Zealand, with the sinking of the ferry 'Wahine', with 734 people on board. The latest broadcasts mentioned that at least 55 lives had been lost. I dearly hoped that none of my family had been involved and was later relieved to find out that this was the case. My heart went out to the families who had lost someone.

That night, we occupied an ambush site that we had used two nights earlier. About midnight, we could hear the sounds of many enemy troops approaching. The noise was so loud that the rest of our squad sleeping away from the ambush site was aroused, and we all prepared to engage with this large enemy force. As they approached, they turned out to be a herd of domestic water buffalo, and they walked through the ambush site. In the dark, I thought I saw several VC walking amongst the herd, but I couldn't be sure. We all held our fire. At our debriefing the next morning, several others also thought they had seen Viet Cong walking in the middle of the herd. "Cunning buggers!" The terse comment summed up all our thoughts.

"When are these bastards going to realise, they are beaten and give up? We have repeatedly kicked their arse the last three months and still they come back for more. I'm fed up!" voiced one guy, reflecting the frustration we all felt.

During one patrol, a member of our squad, bored with the war, and making sure no one was looking, placed an earphone in his ear and plugged it into his transistor radio in the top of his pack. Then he turned the volume to full and lost himself in his own world of rock-and-roll. After a while, the squad paused for a moment, and he absent-mindedly bumped into the man in front of him. He spun his head around to see what was happening, which pulled the earplug cord out of his radio, causing the main speaker to burst into life. Suddenly, the jungle stillness was shattered by the loud voice of Elvis Presley and his band.

"You ain't nothing but a hound dog." Our sharp reflexes caused us all to dive for cover while turning our weapons in his direction, ready to blast the sudden unexpected noise. He stood there frozen in his tracks as he looked down the barrels of seventeen weapons surrounding and trained on him. He quickly dropped his pack and turned off the cause of our fright. Lt. Mountfort marched up to him, seized the radio and led the man away for a stern talking to. The rest of us exchanged smiling glances, or snickered laughter and shook our heads in a mixture of understanding and alarmed at the danger he put us all in. I embarrassingly remembered my own serious mistakes since being in Vietnam.

Midday on the 19th, we returned to Nui Dat with no enemy contacts.

Blue re-joined us from his short prison sentence in Vung Tau. He seemed bitter and changed, but then I supposed we all had.

In our tent I discovered a nest of large black spiders and realised, not for the first time, just how anxious I was towards such creatures. Of all the 'creepy-crawlies' in this jungle, and those in Malaysia, snakes, leeches, scorpions, centipedes, ferocious biting red ants, to name just a few, spiders were what I reviled the most. This feeling was probably the result of my encounter with the tarantula several months earlier. Whatever the reason, I was more than relieved when one guy took charge and removed them.

In the bar that night, I was having a beer with Blue, who was feeling depressed. When I asked him how they had treated him, he replied.

"Not too bad, I guess. But they had ways to make you feel like shit most of the time."

I felt my anger rising.

"I bet those buggers have never even fired a shot in anger, or even seen a bloody VC. I guess it must be hard for them to understand that blokes need to let off steam occasionally. Who has their lives on the line every day? Besides, just because some stupid officer's jaw gets in the way of you innocently, and yes, merrily waving your arms around," I smiled and winked at Blue. Someone else chimed in with:

"They just have no sense of humour at all. And furthermore, people like Blue Neame need to unwind in perhaps more unconventional ways." Everyone at the table laughed and then all started adding their own highly exaggerated methods of how Blue should 'unwind.' The suggestion that got the biggest laugh was:

"How about this one? All the officers line up and Blue goes down the line and, in turn, punches each one. The last one still standing has to take Blue to Vung Tau for a week and pay for all his drinks, meals and, of course, a lady of Blue's choice and act as his servant. But his main job will be to remain standing by, as a willing punching bag, just in case Blue has a need to suddenly punch an officer."

I love the Kiwi humour at such times and was happy to see blue's energy lift as he enjoyed the hilarity.

The jokes against officers were rampant, as they are in most armies throughout the world. But despite the jokes, the officers of V2 Company were highly respected because of their outstanding leadership and courage during combat. The jokes were more about letting off steam than any disrespect towards them.

Graham suddenly appeared at our table and sat down.

"Have you heard the latest? The news from Company HQ is that Whitworth has recommended you, Sas, old boy, for an M.I.D (Mentioned In Despatches) as the result of the last contact."

I was astonished.

"I don't understand. Why me?"

"Looks like it's for bravery in the face of the enemy."

"I can't see why. We all did our bit." I replied.

"Well, I guess it was because you kept your cool, woke everyone up, and let Charlie get in so close before you fired the claymores. That was how we got as many as we did."

"I didn't fire the claymores," I answered. "I was doubtful that they should have been fired at all, because there were so many of them. It was only because a Charlie started climbing the bank that would have revealed our position that someone had the mind to fire them. He's the one who should be decorated, because he was the one who saved all our arses. Who was it now? Was it IB, Mitch or Toy or maybe Dick Dargaville? It was one of those guys."

"Yes, but you could have fired them too early if you'd panicked. And being the strength they were, if the claymores had been prematurely fired, they could very well have over-run us. So, let me buy you a beer. Oh, by the way," he continued as he got up to go to the bar, "Four platoon killed four VC last night. Three of them were women."

Six months later, Sgt. John Whitworth was awarded the M.I.D. for leadership and bravery under fire from this contact. Recommending me for a decoration was typical of the high standard of fine leadership among the Officers and NCOs of V2. Here, John had tried to pass on the recognition to his men, in this case, me. Fortunately, High Command recognised this and rightly so, decorated him with the M.I.D. instead. I felt he deserved it and was glad for him.

Dick Dargaville was to also receive an M.I.D. six months later, not for this incident, but for bravery during the battle on the 7th of February. As a machine gunner, he was under constant fire from an enemy RPG (Rocket propelled grenade launcher) to silence him. Not being able to see where the RPG was, it was so dark; he crawled towards the enemy position and neutralized the enemy RPG section with hand grenades. Then he returned to man his machine gun for the rest of the battle. He should have received an even higher award for his bravery at a key moment when the outcome of the battle could have gone either way.

On the 21st, Six Platoon left Nui Dat for another two-day patrol with ambushes at night. One VC walked through the ambush site on the second night. He got through because we thought others were following him and wanted the maximum number in the ambush before springing it. Had we ambushed the lone VC and an enemy platoon was following, the consequences could have been bad for us. It was not always easy to make snap decisions in such moments.

We returned to Nui Dat at midday on the 23rd, in time to watch an Australian stage show production with female performers. It was more than wonderful, with the performers making great jokes relevant to our situation with strong sexual overtones.

Later that afternoon, they briefed us on our own coming show, the next operation starting on the 25th. This was to be the last operation both for 2 RAR before their return to Australia, and for V2. I was so happy to learn that I was to remain behind and help protect Nui Dat. I had been on every operation so far, and finally it was my turn to remain behind. Perhaps I will survive this madness and see my family again.

I stood looking as V Company lifted off in their Huey's and thundered overhead towards their objective, six platoon leading, followed by the rest of the battalion. I felt the same stirring of excitement that I knew my mates would be feeling at that moment of a simulated cavalry charge. It was strange not being with them, and a part of me wanted to share their experience.

'No, this war is over for me,' I thought as I walked back to our now empty lines. The SLR I carried felt so heavy after my light M16; one of our section members had taken it over, together with the M79 grenade launcher for this operation.

As the air armada disappeared in the distance, I mentally waved. 'Stay safe, guys, for your last operation. Good luck V Company.'

19

'THE SOLDIER HAD TO DIE ...'

I woke up bathed in sweat, feeling totally disoriented and not knowing where I was. It had been that same nightmare that I had been having every night for over a month: seeing myself standing over and looking down at a dead soldier with half of his face having been hideously shot away. In the dream, I would lean closer to have a better look, only to discover to my horror that it was me who was lying there. Then the scene would change. This time I would still lay there but burnt beyond recognition by a napalm bomb. At other times, I had woken from this same nightmare with the first thought that my bed was on fire from having gone to sleep with a lit cigarette in my hand. Some nights I even leapt out of bed and frantically searched through the blankets for the offending fictitious cigarette, only to discover that it had all been a bad dream. Then remembering that I never smoked in bed before sleep. These dreams had been getting steadily worse and was further evidence that I was going crazy.

On April 26th, ten of us who had remained behind from the current operation drove out of Nui Dat in three Land Rovers on a patrol and headed west. We had been assured that there were no enemy units in the area, and it was just a routine patrol. After driving for twenty minutes, we were dropped off and continued on foot. Joe Runga was in command, with Dick Dargaville as lead scout and me as cover scout. The patrol was uneventful as expected, and we routinely set up an ambush that night. The next morning, we pushed on until we arrived at a small stream with high banks, then moved about 300 metres back from it and camped for the day. I told Joe that I needed some water and he replied with.

"While you are at it, just check for any signs of Charlie. You can go on your own. This is a pretty safe area."

"Sure. See you soon."

I moved towards the stream, glad at Joe's reassurance of it being safe. As I approached the riverbank, I found a rough track leading down a steep descent, with a flat open area at the bottom, next to the stream. I noticed that tall and thick vegetation grew almost to the water's edge on the other side of the stream. I felt uneasy. That same old gut-feeling of danger was nagging me. I cautiously pushed my way through some bamboo, then quickly covered the open ground to the water's edge. Something wasn't right, but there was nothing out of place except for what I felt. Slowly stooping down to fill a water bottle, I kept a watchful eye and my rifle trained on the opposite bank. Then I heard the crack of a twig on the other side of the stream, only thirty metres away, and knew instantly what my gut feeling had been trying to tell me. Charlie was in the area. I was a fool for having come alone. Quickly and as quietly as possible, I put my water bottle back into its pouch and looked around for cover, for I was totally exposed. Still looking in the direction where I suspected a VC to be, I quickly retreated to the bamboo cover. In my haste to get back, my boot scraped against a rock, making a noise which I was sure could be heard in Saigon. I silently cursed my clumsiness. Alerted to my whereabouts, someone made a rapid movement to my right, and then silence. I crept to my left, ever watchful for the first glimpse of him. It had to be an enemy because this was a restricted area. Whoever got the first shot in would probably win. I felt excited as we stalked each other. I was not backing down from a perceived unspoken challenge I felt from a VC on the other side of the stream.

I stood on a twig, and the crack caused me to freeze. A full minute passed, not daring to move, when I heard a faint movement from the other side, some distance from where I had thought the VC was. Wow, this guy's good, I thought. Without making the slightest sound, he had moved thirty metres through the very dense undergrowth, bamboo and shingle that lined the river's edge. Both of us were silently moving, hoping to get a glimpse of the other and to fire that first vital shot. It occurred to me to blast the complete area in semi-automatic fire. No, that would really give my position away. I picked up a rock and threw it twenty metres away on my side of the stream, hoping to draw his attention or his fire. It landed with a thud, but no response. This guy was cool, a real professional hunter, with probably as much determination as me. I was about to throw a second rock to the same place, when it occurred to me, he may hear even the slight rustle sound of my clothes as I swung my arm. Also, it was eerily quiet as the usual insect and bird noises had ceased, like in earlier times just before a contact. This further alarmed me. I kept silently and slowly moving, ever seeking a better location than waiting in one place trying to see him, while listening for the slightest sound.

I faintly heard him, and again he was twenty metres away from where I was sure he had been. I let out a long breath and realised I hadn't been breathing at all. The suspense was overwhelming. Fear mingled with excitement, was causing perspiration to trickle down my forehead and into my eyes. My hands were sweaty and shaking slightly. 'Don't crack now, Sas. Your life totally depends upon keeping cool like never before,' I told myself grimly. Nearly 3 and a half years of SAS, and infantry jungle warfare training as well as 6 months of combat experience were what I had to draw on for this, perhaps final climax of my tour. 'I can beat this guy!' An ancient primal hunting urge was taking me over and my only thought was to win.

I sat still for a longer period, waiting to catch the slightest sound, or to see the top of a bush move as he brushed past it. Yes, there he was. I saw the top of a tree move and took careful aim at the tree's base, checking for the twentieth time that the safety catch was off. Suddenly I heard him twenty-five metres away from the moving bush. 'Damn, maybe there are two of them?' No, my senses were too well-tuned; There was only one.

The cat-and-mouse game was now making me worried. My opponent was very skilful. Perhaps he has been fighting in this war for many more years, with much more to draw on than I had. I felt that in the next ten minutes one of us would die, and there was a 50% chance that it would be me. It was a chilling thought. Once again, my life hung in the balance. I was due to leave this country in a fortnight, and I didn't want it to be in a body bag. I felt the absurdity of the situation: two men stalking and trying to kill each other. This was no game, but a deadly serious contest which would end with only one winner. I re-confirmed that the winner would be me. But now, I was sure I knew exactly where he was.

I saw a large rock, slightly to my left, and closer to the water's edge. It offered a better view, and I knew I could see my opponent from there. I picked myself up, and keeping low, sprinted towards it. As I ran, I saw the flash of his AK47 and heard the crack as the rounds passing close over my head. Then I felt a bullet smash through my upper lip, taking teeth, bone, and flesh with it, and pass out the back of my neck. My head was thrust violently backward and was suddenly half lying on my back on my buckled legs. I struggled, drunkenly trying to get back to kneeling upright.

Feeling no pain, and grasping my SLR in one hand by the pistol grip, and unsteadily trying to take aim at where the shots had come from. Before I could press the trigger, I saw the flashes again, felt two bullets tear into my lower gut and doubled over as if I had been kicked in the stomach. The pain in my lower abdomen was agonising. I was crouching on my knees with my face on the stones. Opening my eyes, blood was everywhere. Everything was hazy, and I lifted my head slightly. Large blobs of blood, teeth, bits of bone and gristle were slowly pouring in an endless stream, from half of my mangled face hanging strangely out of place. Knowing I was gravely wounded, everything was growing dim. I rolled onto my side, coughed from breathing blood into my lungs. I saw the outline of a figure dressed in black cautiously approaching me – and slowly passed into blackness.

* * *

I sat bolt upright bathed in sweat, feeling totally disorientated. Panic-stricken, I felt my face and was relieved. Marina held me tightly in her arms and I felt safe as her love and the curves of her body melted into mine. I could not speak and tell her I had just witnessed my own death twenty-four years earlier in Vietnam. The memory of the nightmare surged through my mind like a tornado, causing my body to heave and shake uncontrollably. The pain in my stomach caused me to nearly faint with its intensity, and the blood and bits of my face pouring from my head seemed as real as if it had really happened.

My body at last relaxed and I slumped back onto the bed and curled myself more into Marina's body. I breathed more deeply, allowing myself to fall ever deeper into my subconscious … remembering … allowing the pain and the trauma to be released from my tortured mind and shaking body … remembering what had really happened all those years ago.

* * *

I looked across to the other side of the stream, while the sweat dripped off the end of my nose. My enemy was waiting and watching for his chance. My rifle was wet with the sweat from my hands and my concentration was interrupted as perspiration dripped into my eyes. Carefully, while still holding my rifle in the aiming position with my right hand, I untied my black scarf around my neck. Removing my hat, then tied the scarf around my head as a sweatband.

Something was happening that I didn't understand. It was like 'deja vu.' Throughout the last two days: us driving out of Nui Dat in three Land Rovers, checking the river, and for the last fifteen minutes stalking a deadly enemy, was as if I'd lived out this sequence of my life somewhere before. As I threw the rock to draw his attention and got no response, I felt like I was acting in a re-run of a rehearsed stage production. Perhaps I really am going crazy! The conversation in my head was becoming desperate, as if trying to work something out of vital importance. I pinched myself to see if I wasn't dreaming, but my confusion remained. My gut feeling seemed like it was warning me that something terrible was going to happen. But I was too confused with the flashes of past, present, and future experiences all happening at the same time and the mounting fear growing in my stomach.

I stopped moving and sat still for several minutes, rifle aimed, waiting to catch the slightest sound from him, or to see the top of a bush move as he passed it. This guy is a real professional, I thought. In the next ten minutes, I felt that one of us would die, and there was a 50% chance that it would be me. Even Russian roulette has better odds. That thought brought me back to my senses. This is crazy, and if this is stupid, then all bloody war is stupid. But, from the last slight sound he had made, I was sure I knew where he was.

Suddenly I saw a large rock slightly to my left, close to the water's edge on my side. I knew I would be able to see him from there. I picked myself up and prepared to sprint towards it.

My mind exploded with the gruesome image of a dead New Zealand soldier with most of his face blown away. There was a brief, stabbing pain in my stomach and I sat down again.

'What the hell is happening to me? I will not survive with this confusion. I need all my senses and I don't have them.'

I checked in on how I was feeling. I was totally afraid and sensed that I was in extreme danger, perhaps worse than ever before in my life. Keeping an eye on where my adversary might be, I focused inside on my feelings, which I intuitively felt I could trust. First came more fear and as I was fully present with it, it changed to an acceptance of what is in the here and now!

This acceptance triggered the similar altered state to when caught in the ambush. Now, as before, I felt this enormous, gentle interest in everything around me. Again, that incredible sensation of pure happiness flowed throughout my entire body. There seemed to be no sense of time or motion. My breathing was gentle, relaxed, with no stress in my body. It was the freest I had ever felt. 'I'm not going crazy,' I concluded. In fact, this was the sanest moment I had ever felt.

How long I sat there, I will never know. Finally, the intense joyful feeling subsided, replaced by a gentle, loving state. My heart went out to my brother across the other side of the stream, who I sensed was still there.

"Stay safe, my friend. I'm going home."

Knowing that I could never kill again, but also that an immediate danger still existed. I looked around for a safe retreat, because if he got even the slightest glimpse of me, his shot may not miss. Seeing a small dried out waterway leading down from the top of the bank, I slowly crawled to it. Yes, it would hide me from view. Then rolled onto my back, and out of habit, keeping my rifle trained on the opposite bank, pushed myself upward with my legs. If he suddenly appeared, I would put a shot above him so he would be forced to keep his head down.

My efforts to crawl backwards up the bank were noisy and would have been heard by him, but I was confident he couldn't see me. I could faintly hear him moving, trying to get his sights on me. A full ten minutes later, on reaching the top, I rested from the effort of the awkward and exhausting backward climb. I could still sense him down there and fervently hoped he would survive the war. Once clear of the river, I hurried back to where the squad was resting and reported.

"Charlie's in the area, and I think we should leave."

"Okay, pack up everyone," Joe unhesitatingly retorted. "We'll move to another area, establish a camp, then we'll come back and do a sweep,"

Two hours later, we did a sweep of the stream, but my personal adversary had long gone, probably to warn his comrades of my presence. We put in an ambush that night nearby, but much to my relief, the VC had been warned out of the area. The next morning, we patrolled all the way back to Nui Dat, arriving at midday.

The following day I stood looking out of my tent at the first rain of the coming monsoon season. Water was pouring incessantly off the tent sides and trickling down the holding ropes. My thoughts became mingled with the trickling water. What happened out there two days ago? Vaguely, I remembered a river and crawling around as if my life depended on it. My usual nightmare of being shot through the face happened again last night, but even though it was very vivid, it was much less intense emotionally, as if I had released something. Somehow, there seemed to be a connection between this dream and what happened two days ago. But I was at a loss for what it might be. As I thought about that event, it all seemed more like a distant dream than reality, and it was difficult to figure out between the two. Perhaps one day I may understand what really happened out there beside that stream. One day, I may even understand what I am doing here in Vietnam. Right now, I sure as hell do not. I left the page of the date from 2 days ago blank and would complete it if my memory of it ever returned.

Two days later, ten of us made up a squad for another four-day patrol South of Nui Dat. Our mission was to find any VC units moving through the area. With only ten more days to go in Vietnam, life had never been more precious. It seemed like our leadership was keeping us busy so as not to dwell on the approaching completion of our tour. Fortunately, the patrol was uneventful, though we had an alarming encounter on our return.

We were patrolling in open formation, five men in an extended line, with a second line following the first at about 30 metres behind. We were sweeping the ground for hidden enemy bunkers, footprints, or any other enemy signs. I was in the second line, acting as cover. Suddenly, we disturbed the largest king cobra snake I had ever seen. On seeing us, the snake quickly slithered away towards the guys in the forward section, who had already passed it by unnoticed. John Dallow, in our group, saw it first and gave a warning shout.

"Look out, Blue, a snake coming in your direction."

Blue turned, his eyes searching the ground around him. They saw each other at the same time, only one metre apart. The cobra reared up to strike, its hood fully extended on either side of its head, a terrifying sight. Without taking a step back, Blue levelled his M60 and fired. The bullets struck the snake's body, hurling it to the ground but not killing it. As the cobra raised up prepared to strike again, Blue calmly fired another burst and knocked it down again. Once more, the snake rose and struck out ferociously. Blue fired yet again with deadly accuracy and with the coolness he had always displayed in battle. For the third time, bullets cut into the cobra and finally, wounded, the creature retreated and disappeared down a hole.

We all stood dumbfounded at what we had just seen. "Bloody hell! Nice one, Blue," someone called out. Blue just smiled and, without comment, turned to continue the sweep as if nothing had happened. That was so typical of him.

On May 10, 1968, V2 company returned to Nui Dat from its operation. For the first time, I was not interested in how many kills they had made. Someone told me the number, and it was a lot. I was more interested if any of our guys had been hurt, which unfortunately there had been five wounded from 4 platoon.

The next week passed quickly and was mostly spent in packing and saying goodbye to Australian 'cobber's' (friends) and to our own mates in W Company.

The lone plane dropped slowly out of the sky and landed. It was a Bristol freighter, the pride of the New Zealand Airforce, and a relic of the Second World War. An American bystander scratched his head. "My God, the Wright Brothers have landed!"

"No way, Yank," Danny McPhail quickly answered.

"That's New Zealand's latest secret weapon that you probably haven't heard about." We all laughed, including the American.

As I stepped aboard the freighter, I paused and turned round for my last look at Vietnam. A lone Huey flew overhead; the yellow and red striped flag fluttered over the ARVN post near the entrance to Vung Tau airbase; US and Australian personnel went about their business. Nothing had changed since we had arrived six months earlier. Yet, everything had changed for the men who climbed aboard that aircraft. The thoughts and feelings of what seemed like many lifetimes, all crammed into six months, flooded through me, and I felt a tear on my cheek. It was the only one I ever shed on my tour. Even in my worst moments, I had never allowed myself the luxury of such an emotion. I quickly wiped the tear away, turned and stepped into the plane.

As the Bristol freighter lifted off and headed towards Singapore, I wrote the last words in my diary, "Goodbye Charlie, Nui Dat, the killing, and Vietnam. Goodbye Vietnam. Signed: PTE. C.P. SISSON. May 14, 1968." I then wrapped it in a brown paper bag. It was to be 24 years later before I opened it. Little did I know that, as a 'wounded warrior', the nightmare had barely begun, still holding onto many of the horrific memories to which I thought I had just bid farewell to. But the healing had begun.

The soldier in me had to die, to make way for the rebirth of the peaceful, emotional warrior.

A soldier's song: Written by Max Gawler, V2 company, after many years of his own personal healing process.

"When I was young, yes, young and single, I served my country and went to war.
It was to be a great adventure. Didn't really know what we were fighting for.
Go kill the commies, that's what they told us, make the world

a better place.
But I was soon to realise that, in every war there is a human face.
I've seen the killing and the dying. I've seen the maiming and the fear,
And in the midst of the confusion, would ask myself, 'what am I doing here?'
So, here we are so many years onward, and fine young men still go to war.
And like my father and fathers before him, I'm still wondering what it was really for…"

20
MALAYSIA

"It's so quiet," I said to Colin, who was dozing beside me. Being 2 a.m. and the bus was dark, with most of the guys dozing. I was struck by the absence of the constant, distant rumbling sound of artillery fire to which we had become accustomed to, for the last six months. We were parked at Singapore Airport, waiting for our papers to be cleared before driving to Terendak camp, just out of Malacca, on the west coast of the Malaysian peninsula.

Terendak, where we were to be for the next six months, was the Southeast Asia British brigade group of four battalions: English, Australian, Gurkhas, and New Zealanders. It was good to see old friends again on our arrival.

On my first leave two days later, I took a taxi into Malacca to visit a young Chinese girlfriend, Susie, whom I'd met two months before leaving for Vietnam. As I was driven into the city, it excited me at the prospect of seeing her again, as well as her young child of two years. I climbed the staircase leading to her apartment. It was just as old and rundown as I remembered it, but seeing her was all that mattered. On reaching the top, I knocked on her door, holding the flowers and chocolates I had bought for her behind my back. No answer. I knocked louder and was puzzled, as I knew she was always there at this time of the day. Several minutes passed, then the door across the hall opened and her girlfriend, whom I knew, came out.

"What are you doing here? You must go from here, quickly." She said with fear on her face.

"Where's Susie? Is she okay?"

The young woman was pulling my arm, nearly dragging me to the staircase.

"Susie dead. Killed by Chinese secret society. You in great danger coming here. Please leave." I staggered under her words.

"What happened? What happened to her child?"

"No time to explain, you must go now." The look of fear in her eyes was the same that I'd seen in men's eyes just before battle, and I knew she was serious. Suddenly sensing that I really was in danger and being unarmed, I thrust the gifts into her hands and bolted down the stairs and out to the safety of the street. After walking aimlessly in shock for several hours, I found a bar and sat there for the rest of the day and, late into the night, getting drunk. I felt totally abandoned, as if I'd been deserted by the entire world. I nearly cried, but I couldn't allow such an emotion.

"Life is so bloody cheap. Why do you let people get killed in this godforsaken country?" My slurred voice made little impact on the Chinese barman who was half asleep and waiting for me to leave, so that he could close at such a late hour. I felt a mixture of sadness, mostly self-pity and anger, as if the violence had followed me from Vietnam. I knew she had some dealings with the Chinese secret society, which was a criminal organization that dealt in drugs, blackmail, prostitution and now, as it seems, murder. Wracking my brain trying to work out what she must have done to merit such a retribution. I wondered what possibly happened to her young daughter, who was the prettiest little girl that I had taken a shine to. That thought made me feel even worse. I don't remember how I got back to camp, but fortunately, woke up the next morning in my bed.

The army, it seemed, didn't know what to do with us. After weeks of leave, which I spent mostly in Singapore, they tried to give us lectures on weapon stripping. I felt sorry for the instructors, as we had stripped such weapons in the dark during battle, almost in our sleep. We didn't hold back in being vocal and showing our distaste and boredom at the instructor's lack of experience. Next, they had us gardening, cleaning weapons, clearing jungle on the edge of camp, or doing whatever else they could think of to keep us occupied. We were uncooperative, ill-disciplined, and belligerent. It showed how easily and quickly it took to transform highly disciplined combat veterans to a low morale, disruptive rabble through the lack of effective leadership. On looking back, I can appreciate that the poor commanders who had been put in charge of us were very lenient, tolerant, and even sympathetic to how we were feeling, but did not know how to treat us. They represented authority and, to confused, angry veterans fresh from a war zone, they became the enemy.

Most nights found us in the local bars, just outside the main entrance to

Terendak camp, where we all drank heavily. Afterwards, we would stagger home, singing Vietnamese and Malaysian songs, praising the glories of the great New Zealand soldier, and having the occasional fight. One night when I walked into a bar looking for the guys, Blue, in his drunken state, mistook me for an Australian entering a predominantly Kiwi bar and knocked me clean out with one powerful punch. 'Those were the days …'

The war in Vietnam, ground on with news reports coming over Malaysian television most nights, was generally repetitive with little good news. Though I was interested in current world affairs, I would walk out, or switch the TV off, whenever any news of Vietnam came on, and particularly whenever any combat scenes were shown. I just could not bring myself, not even for a second, to be reminded of the pain inside me.

Wounded warrior status, more commonly known as PTSD (Post Traumatic Stress Disorder), takes many forms. These include alcohol and drug addiction, domestic violence, and anti-social behaviour, just to name a few. Mine, which is the most common, came as a drastic loss of self-confidence, self-esteem, and a neediness for love and approval. This deep insecurity was to plague my life for the next twenty years. It was finally healed by Breath Integration.

I was missing Susie and a woman's touch. But in reality, I was simply emotionally needy. My eye was caught one evening by an attractive young Chinese girl working in one of the bars. She was very attentive and kind whilst serving our drinks and I couldn't stop myself from falling in love with her, which was really falling in need. Her caring showed me how desperately I needed affection. I would sit in the bar every night and watch her work; it was lovesickness at its worst. I refused to sleep with her, believing her to be at least a princess and above any such casual liaisons. She was a bar girl, and probably a prostitute as well, as most of the bar girls were, but to me she was the divine representation of love, my Don Quixote's, Dulcinea. One afternoon, I invited her to the movies in Malacca just to be close to her. Not knowing beforehand that it was a war movie, and towards the end, I reacted uncontrollably angrily. I remember her looking wide eyed at some things I was heatedly saying. After that incident, she avoided me, and I am sure that my later appearances in the bar caused her embarrassment amongst her friends, and I became the brunt of jokes with my own mates.

One evening, while I was on guard duty at the entrance to our battalion lines, a truck drove through with all my mates returning from a night of drinking in the bars. Rodger Haworth in the back saw me and shouted out drunkenly,

"Hey Sas, we all slept with your little Chinese girlfriend tonight. She's a bloody good root. You want to try it with her sometime."

The truck sped off with a roar of laughter trailing behind. I stood there, knowing they were joking with good nature, but I felt foolish and depressed. My regular visits to the bar where she worked had to stop, as she had no interest in me. I was heartbroken.

A month later, Colin Burgering and I spent a week on the island of Penang, 300 kilometres north of Malacca. On our second day there, I saw an exquisite Malaysian girl serving in a shop. After introducing myself, I asked her if she would go with me for a meal after her work. She agreed, so Colin and I spent the rest of the afternoon swimming and filling in the time before meeting her.

While lying on the beach, listening to an English-speaking Malaysian station on my transistor radio, came the news:

"We interrupt this programme to announce that the Soviet Union has, from last night, launched an invasion into Czechoslovakia. Russian tanks have entered Prague and the loss of life has been reported to be high. There have been many arrests and resistance in much of the city continues but is being steadily overcome by Soviet troops. We will keep you updated as news comes to hand. We return you to our programme …"

Shocked, I looked at Colin.

"Those bloody Russian bastards."

"You know, Sas, the Allies in Vietnam should stop pissing about. They should thrust north, take Hanoi, and keep going through China, and not stop 'till they hit Moscow."

"That might be taking on a bit much," I replied. "But whatever happens, that bloody Soviet Union has got to be stopped. After all, they are behind the war in Vietnam and the Vietnamese people are puppets to the Soviet Union."

I really believed this then, and years later, this was proved untrue.

"Well, we did our bit, Sas."

"Not enough, it seems." I felt a burning anger that day against Russia and would have gladly signed on, had a war resulted from the Czech invasion.

That evening, I fell in love again. The need for female companionship was really the need for a mother. Azizah was more than charming. Her beautiful, dark flashing eyes and very attractive figure made her irresistible. Her nature was soft, and she instinctively fell into a mother's role by stroking my emotional need. Colin had two more days leave, and mine was about to finish and needed to travel back to Terendak the next day. Instead, I decided to go AWOL (absence without leave) to stay on with Colin and enjoy this blooming romance with Azizah for two extra days. Within twelve hours of my transgression, I had been reported and was arrested by the local British Military Police. However, I was able to talk on the phone to our orderly officer back in Terendak and convinced him I would return on the next available flight. He spoke to the MPs and was released for another twenty-four hours of bliss. They dropped the serious charge of AWOL on my return; because of our regimental police being so tolerant towards the veterans. Such a serious charge would have cost me a jail term in normal circumstances.

I signed up with 30 others on a tiger safari in north Malaysia for ten days. We split up into teams of five men and travelled mainly by boat in deep jungle rivers to remote locations in North Malaysia.

It was a wonderful trip, but my heart was back in Penang. We shot no tigers, in which years later I was glad about with these magnificent creatures. In 1968, tigers were not an endangered species, and the Malaysian government permitted hunting them under licence.

We travelled first by land rovers and then by boats up rivers through jungle probably never seen by Europeans, except during the Malayan emergency against the Communists fifteen years earlier. It was thick with wild game, especially wild pigs and plentiful with tigers. The area was also full of leeches, even away from water, unlike in Vietnam. It was our only unpleasant encounter.

What struck me most was the delightful character of the local people we met along the way. In Malacca, I had not been over-impressed with some Malaysians, partly because I met them mostly in bars, not the best environment to meet genuine people. By contrast, the people in the kampongs, (jungle villages) were a gentle and genuine people. The thought crossed my mind, as the boat carried us up a long, narrow river on our way to 'tiger country', was to desert the Army, then fetch Azizah and return to live with them. Only the memory of my family back home stopped me. It didn't occur to me that Azizah probably would have had some objections to giving up a comfortable city life to suddenly live in the leech infested jungle. I was emotionally unstable living a romantic Don Quixote fantasy.

After arriving at a remote location and set up a camp, and just at dusk, we saw a leopard in the distance. It was such a beautiful and majestic creature that I decided I could never again shoot any living thing.

On our return to Terendak, I applied for more leave and flew up to

Penang. I cut down on my drinking to be with Azizah and our time together was wonderful. She worked most days, so I spent the time sightseeing around the island. One day, I met up with some Australians from Terendak and fell into an intense drinking bout with them. I told them I had to be at a certain place to meet Azizah, as we had planned to go to the very best Chinese restaurant in Penang, and they promised, no matter what, they'd ensure that I got there. By late afternoon, though, I was very drunk and could barely stand. At the allotted hour, my Aussie mates put me in a taxi where I passed out. When I next opened my eyes, Azizah was standing outside the taxi, and was far from happy at my appearance. I'll never know how this taxi found her because I had told no one where we were to meet.

"Would you prefer to go back to the hotel rather than go out?" she asked, hiding her initial annoyance.

"No, let's go to the restaurant." I slurred. "I promised you a really good dinner and I haven't eaten all day."

Later, sitting in the beautifully decorated restaurant, I felt the effects of my all-day drinking. I was suddenly ill in the restaurant and ran to the men's room to clean myself up. I felt so embarrassed that I had made such an idiot of myself in front of Azizah. I concluded she would never want to see me again. Leaving the restaurant by the rear exit, without a word to her, I walked down to the waterfront, feeling deeply sorry for myself. I sat there for an hour, chain-smoking and cursing the state of my life.

"Colin! Are you okay?" Azizah's gentle and concerned voice reached me from out of the darkness.

"How did you find me? Oh, that doesn't matter. I'm so dreadfully sorry, and I'm feeling so terrible at what happened that I ..."

She placed her finger over my lips to silence me. "I love you, dear man." I looked into her beautiful dark eyes that invited what I most needed, love and security. At that moment, the moon above us, the sound of the waves, and Azizah's comforting arms around me, I quietly asked: "Azizah, will you marry me, and come with me to New Zealand?"

She looked at me in astonishment. "Goodness me, Colin," she exclaimed. "We have only been with each other for little over seven days. But I love you and so, yes."

On my return to camp, my application to take Azizah back to New Zealand was turned down because she was a Moslem, and in 1968 there were no places for Moslems to worship back home. The orderly officer explained the Army was not prepared to use taxpayers' money to take a young Moslem out of her natural environment.

"Okay then. I'll get out of this damn Army and go back for her." I angrily replied. The officer leaned forward over his desk.

"You do that, Sisson, but let me give you a word of advice. These Asian women might be beautiful when they're young, but by thirty they're old women. And besides, they don't think like us, particularly Moslems. Their culture is so different, you'll have many problems."

I could barely contain my anger.

"Thank you, *sir,* but with all due respect, I think they are your prejudices. Am I dismissed?"

A few days later, the remaining personnel in the now dissolved V2 Company, who had not returned to New Zealand, held a dance. Around midnight, three of us took a taxi into Malacca and check out the local action. After visiting several bars, we met up with four fellow Kiwis. One of them handed me a thunderflash and suggested we all go down to the Malaccan waterfront where there were some ancient Portuguese cannons, stick the thunderflash in one of them, and fire it. We all agreed and, being a little drunk by this stage, wobbled down to where the cannons were. But we couldn't get the striker on the thunderflash to work, so after many attempts, I placed it in my back pocket, with the intention to later discard it. Most of the guys went looking for a taxi to go back to camp, leaving three of us to spend more time enjoying Malacca. After about an hour, we decided it was time for us to head home as well.

"What happened to that thunderflash?" Frank* asked me.

"It doesn't work. Here, take it," I answered, handing it to him. He looked at it, and to test it, pulled the striker. It hissed into life. We looked at each other, amused and surprised that it works after all. Frank threw it quickly into a storm drain. The explosion, accentuated by the confined space in the drain, must have been heard throughout much of Malacca. I looked up and saw that we were standing right outside the Hong Kong Shanghai bank.

"Bloody hell, let's get out of here."

To set off an explosion outside a major bank was bad enough, but most of Malaysia was on a military alert by the conflict with Indonesia. Occasionally, Indonesian commandos raided cities on the coast close to Indonesia, in which Malacca was situated. Such an explosion would trigger many police and military quick response units within the vicinity.

We ran off down a side street, around a corner, right into the arms of

---

* *Frank was not his real name due to sensitivity of the situation.*

a pistol-waving Malaysian police officer, who was running to the scene of the explosion. Frank put his hands up while the two of us ran off. I went down a dark alley that led nowhere. Eventually I joined up with my other friend and went looking for Frank, whom we saw was being led off to the police station at gunpoint.

"Let's rescue him and get back to camp."

We sprinted after them, not at all sure how we were to carry out such a mission. Being quite drunk rarely allows for rational thinking at such crucial moments. We had nearly caught up with them when a truck with a dozen police in the back, pulled round the corner. On seeing us, quickly disembarked. Having been called out in the emergency following the explosion, most were carrying sub-machine guns. They surrounded us, whereupon my friend looked enquiring at me as if to ask whether we should take them on. Looking down the menacing barrels of so many sten submachine guns, we decided to surrender and go with them, quietly.

After being taken to the police station, they separated us in separate cells out of view or hearing range of each other. Each one of us, in turn, was questioned. On my turn, was led into a small office and sat in a chair. One of the officers adjusted a spotlight onto my face and I burst out laughing. Remembering the counter interrogation training in the SAS, I was highly amused by their amateur approach.

"Don't you 'buggers' know that they only use an interrogation spotlight in Hollywood movies?" I sneered.

The two police sergeants conversed angrily in Malay, which I couldn't understand. Suddenly, their boss arrived, and they had a one-minute conference. Then the two sergeants roughly pulled me out of the chair by the scruff of the neck, threw me against the wall and stingingly slapped my face several times, but not hard enough to draw blood. My belligerence and drink-induced bravado quickly melted. They then angrily half-dragged me to a small tin shed, with one set of iron bars covering a small window, at the back of the station. They roughly threw me inside and locked the door. I crawled onto and fell asleep on the rough boards of a bed, hearing a rat scuttle across the bare, uneven, wet concrete floor. I woke the next morning, extremely thirsty after a night of alcohol. At my repeated request, the police refused me a drink. As the sun rose, the shed heated up, but still no drink was forthcoming. By four o'clock in the afternoon, with my head pounding and tongue swollen, I was relieved to see two members of our own military police arrive and saw one of them had been in Vietnam with us. He took one look at me and went back inside the main office, where I heard raised voices in argument about the way I had been treated. The three of us were released and driven away, towards Terendak. The MP vehicle stopped at the first shop we came to, and our rescuers bought three large soft drinks that tasted like Heaven.

Over the next two weeks, we were interrogated by the British CID (Central Investigation Division). They were convinced, as had been the Malaysian police, that we had tried to blow our way into the bank. Because of my demolition training in the SAS, made me the chief suspect.

"Well, Sisson. You might as well admit it. The other two have, and both say on sworn oath that all three of you had planned to break into the bank, and that you used high explosives to do so."

I knew this to be a mere ploy, recognising the similar interrogation training I'd had as this officer.

"Is that right, sir? I repeat, my name is Private Sisson, and my regimental number is … and I am innocent of all charges of attempted bank robbery."

"Come now, Colin."

He was now using the friendly approach to win my confidence and weaken my resolve.

"You're not in the SAS now, and you haven't been captured by the enemy. We're just here to help. Just tell us the truth, and you will get a light sentence, due to your war service in Vietnam. I will recommend extra leniency if you cooperate."

"I repeat. My name is private Sisson, registration number…."

The officer coldly looked at me, his face expressionless, and tried to stare me out. I sat there staring back, gripped with him in a battle of wills, neither refusing to surrender. Finally, with the slight hint of a smile, he said. "You're a stubborn bastard, aren't you? Okay, corporal, take him away, and bring in the next one."

The interrogation sessions happened five times that first day, but less for my other two friends. The following three days, they grilled me three times each day. It was a gruelling time and was grateful for my SAS training. I learned a lot from having the live experience of interrogation at first hand. The remains of the thunderflash were never found to back up our story, presumably having been washed away.

Our ordeal finally ended two weeks later when one of the others finally cracked and admitted that he had tried to break into the bank. Frank felt guilty at seeing his mate charged and so also made a false confession. I refused to give in and was finally released. At the court martial hearing several weeks later, I was called as a prime witness, but even during the hearing, the CID officer tried to get me to confess in front of the court that it was me who had set off the explosion. Because of my training with explosives, I felt everyone in that room was equally convinced I was guilty. My two friends got twenty-one days in prison for something they hadn't done. It was a light sentence for attempted bank robbery because of their excellent war records. We exchanged glances as they were led away after the judgement.

On leaving the court, the British CID sergeant, who had been helping throughout the investigation, came up to me.

"You bastard, letting your friends take the rap for you. We both know it was you who set off the explosive charge."

"Well, sergeant," I sneered, "It looks like I really cheated the law this time."

On my next leave, I went back to Penang. There was a severe cholera epidemic on the island, so it was closed to outsiders. However, after producing documents to prove I had all my vaccination shots, I was allowed entry.

Azizah and I became formally engaged. Problems arose when she insisted that I would have to become a Moslem. I knew her religion was very dear to her, but I thought of a way to persuade her to have a Christian wedding. Knowing the Moslem male tradition in Malaysia, I suggested to her.

"Okay. I'll become a Moslem on the condition that I can have four wives."

"Alright," she answered, calling my bluff, "As long as I am the first."

Little did I realise that in Islamic lore there is a special honour in being the first wife. We put this sensitive subject to one side, hoping the problem would eventually sort itself out. I secretly hoped that she would change her mind on her arrival in New Zealand, when she would be exposed to my culture and religion.

Our time together was wonderful until the fourth day, when I felt intense cramps in my stomach and had severe diarrhoea and a throbbing headache. I woke up vomiting in the middle of the night. The stomach cramps and diarrhoea became as intense as my bout of dysentery in Vietnam. I could barely move and asked Azizah to phone the doctor back in Terendak camp. After an hour, she finally reached him at 2 a.m. She described the symptoms and informed him of the cholera epidemic. By this time, I was convinced I had the disease.

"It sounds a bit like it, but I don't think he has that. I'll get his records out in the morning. Can you get him on a plane first thing tomorrow morning? I'm sure he doesn't have cholera, but as a safety precaution, don't let him touch anyone, nor tell the airlines he is sick. They may not let him off the island if they suspect he has something."

This conversation that was relayed to me afterwards was no comfort to my fears. Azizah was clearly worried about me. I got an early morning flight back to Kuala Lumpur, where an ambulance from Terendak was waiting for me.

"You bloody idiot Sisson." I was sitting on the bed in the regimental aid post, feeling terrible, while the doctor checked my medical records. "Why didn't you check in here with me on your return from Vietnam? It looks like you're got a severe relapse of dysentery. In fact, you've had it all the time, but it was suppressed with the drugs you took while there. Don't you know you can die from this disease? I'm furious at you and you are off to hospital."

I have no recollection of the next three days, as I lapsed into a coma. On the fourth day, I finally woke, attached to a drip, feeling like my body was disintegrating. I could barely move and had to be helped to release the blood-laden filth from my bowels.

Some New Zealanders, also patients in the hospital, discovered I was there and brought me reading material. To my delight, I woke up one afternoon to find a TV that they had appropriated from the TV room, positioned at the end of my bed. I enjoyed television for four hours until the hospital staff located the 'lost' set and had it returned. My new comrades, whose kindness I'll never forget, later stole back the TV on several occasions and an amusing power struggle ensued between my new friends and the hospital staff.

After fourteen days, I improved and noticed a European woman in my ward. This was a particular pleasure, as I had not seen a European woman for nearly two years. Barbara was an Australian sister, sadly for me already engaged, who was especially kind to me. She had a brother who had served with 7 RAR in Vietnam, of whom she was very fond, and perhaps because of this, paid me special attention. True to tradition, I soon fell madly in love with my nurse, and have no doubt that my passion for her was a major factor in my excellent recovery progress. Knowing that 'Barbara' was spoken for, I never shared my 'undying' love with her, but I began to think about my commitment to Azizah. Was it perhaps merely an infatuation that I felt for her? Slowly and painfully, I was realising how damaged, needy, and vulnerable my feelings were. In fact, it was now becoming alarmingly obvious to me that if a door handle were to give me some affection, I would fall in love with it! But it was not love for someone, but the need to be loved that I craved. A hurt child's perspective and a clear sign of a wounded warrior.

Knowing however hard it might be for both of us, it was a time for total honesty, if I could manage such a thing.

"Dear Azizah," I wrote. "My illness has given me many insights into my relationship with you, and I have a lot of reservations about it working out between us. I would like to think that I really do love you, but I'm unsure of anything anymore. I truly am sorry, but I see I am not good for you, or probably anyone. Please don't hate me too much, but I must say goodbye."

I never heard back from her, and over the years have often wondered how she lived out her life and how different my life would have been with her. Every day is a crossroads determined only by our choices and decisions we make. Does fate play any part in it? Who knows?

I was on light duties for several weeks after my release from three weeks in hospital. My bowels had been severely damaged and became a weak point: giving me mild diarrhoea for the next twenty years whenever I became emotionally stressed.

My family in New Zealand were eagerly anticipating my return home, and my mother sent me a letter tape with a recording of the song, 'The Green, Green Grass of Home'. This I would play over and over, increasing my excitement. I wondered if they would march us down Queen Street in Auckland when we got home. Such an imagined scene: the Vietnam hero's receiving a rapturous response, with bands playing, banners flying, marching girls ... I smiled at the thought but felt that just to get home would be more than enough.

As soon as I was feeling stronger, I went for short runs and started weightlifting. Then I started spending much of my time working out with an Australian friend, Mike Didman, in Tae Kwon Do, a Korean martial art. My physical recovery was rapid, and, by November, I could board a plane, bound for home.

21

THE GREEN, GREEN GRASS OF HOME

The C-130 aircraft touched down at Whenuapai airbase, just out of Auckland. We disembarked excitedly, then went through customs and paraded. I could see my mother, my sister Adrienne and young brother Grant, standing and waving on the edge of the field.

An officer called us to attention and gave us our final instructions. His words confused us.

"After you are dismissed, join your families and friends, and get out of your uniform as quickly as possible. There's a strong anti-Vietnam-war feeling here in New Zealand. So don't be too vocal about where you have been, particularly when you're with certain groups. Stay out of trouble and report back for duty in four weeks as laid down in your documents. Attention. Dis-miss."

Colin Burgering, standing next to me, glanced in my direction. "What sort of welcome home was that?"

"I don't know. Anyway, come and meet my mum," I replied.

If our initial feelings were of disillusionment and disappointment from our official welcome home, were soon eclipsed by the joy of reuniting with our loved ones after two years. The changes in my family were clear, particularly in my sister and younger brother, who had grown so much. The changes that my family saw in me must have been just as obvious, but out of consideration, they made no comment. My greatest joy was to hold my mother in my arms. Both of us, after our first hug, had to wipe away our tears. She cried openly, both from the happiness of our reunion and from the sadness and pain of our long separation. Coupled with the anxiety of the news reports from Vietnam during the heaviest of fighting must have been terrible for any mother to endure. The dam of tears within me nearly broke as her body heaved with each deep sob, and I only with great effort suppressed the depth of my own feelings.

When we arrived home, the lovely strains of 'The Green, Green Grass of Home' welcomed me. Anyone less inhibited would have broken down in a torrent of tears, but not me. I had to rein in all my willpower just to handle what I felt.

We spent our first evening talking quietly, catching up on two years of lost news and happenings, and sharing gifts. I stayed mainly with my Malaysian experiences, unsure what to say about Vietnam, and equally unsure about what I felt.

Charlie, my stepfather, who had married Mum fifteen years earlier, had seen action in the Libyan desert and in Italy during the Second World War was silently comforting. He never asked me about my experiences in combat, or talked about his own, but there was an unspoken understanding of the hardships and horrors we had both been through. After chatting for a while, he looked long and hard at me, nodded, got up, and went to make a cup of tea. As he did so, a flow of warmth and understanding passed between us. Charlie had always been a wonderful second father to me, but never more so than in that precious moment.

I was missing Azizah, her gentle nature, her soothing touch, and her beautiful dark eyes, but knew that chapter in my life had closed forever. I looked out at the city lights of Auckland from the lounge window. 'Somewhere out there is my future wife. May I find her soon,' I thought. Mum came up to me and stood behind me and wrapped her comforting arms around me.

"Welcome home, son. I'd like you to know that whatever's going on inside you, I'm always here for you. You don't have to talk about anything. Just know that you are safe here at home. I choked back a sob, turned around and held her close to me, fighting back the tears that demanded expression. She cried for both of us, while inviting me that, if I wanted to, it was okay to cry, too.

Her assurance was in vain, for I had a deeply rooted belief that, if I were to survive, I had to keep my feelings under control.

We spent the next day shopping and sightseeing in Auckland. While walking along the street, a car suddenly backfired a common occurrence in cars back in the 1960s. The next I knew, I was looking out at Mum from underneath a parked car. She was staring at me, with her head tilted to one side, with an astonished look on her face.

"Are you all right, Colin?" I pulled myself from under the car, stood up, and brushed the dust from my jacket. I smiled weakly at her and at several curious people passing by.

"Sure, just keeping my reactions in trim," was all I could think of.

Cecil Poa

Years later, I met up with Cecil Poa, who served with 5 platoon, and shared his cultural war experience and homecoming with me.

"As I prepared to head back to camp after my last leave before travelling overseas, I said my goodbyes to my family and the very last person was my grandfather, who was my mentor but more importantly, my kaumatua (elder). It shocked me when he walked away as I extended my hand for a handshake to be followed by a 'hongi.' He uttered the following words of farewell.

"Ma te wa moko, ka kite ano." When translated means:

"All in good time, grandson. I will see you again." As I learned later, it was his way of wishing for my safe return. How did he know that in April of the following year (1967) New Zealand infantry troops would start deploying to Vietnam?

Another experience was that many enemy combatants killed were buried after a contact, unlike other allies, who left them where they fell. This followed the Māori kaupapa (protocol) of returning them to 'Papatuanuku' (mother earth).

Finally, on my return to NZ, one crucial cultural element was missing, and that was the cleansing of the soul, and the spirit called the "whaka noa." This involved lifting off the negative elements of being at war and returning harmony to the 'wairua' (spirit) for me this was not done until 40 years after my return, in 2008. This was a major healing for me and probably didn't happen sooner because I was finally ready for it when it happened." Cecil.

Six months after leaving Vietnam, probably along with Cecil and most of V2 Company, I was still having nightmares about the war, but by that time I could suppress any screams at the moment I woke. This self-control saved me from having to make embarrassing explanations to my concerned family about the state of my mental health.

After four days of relaxation, I travelled south by train to my hometown, Levin, to re-join my father and two older brothers, Warwick and Robin. Dad hugged me strongly as I jumped from the train. All my old friends, brothers and their wives were there to greet me. It was a moving moment, with much shouting and laughing and everyone wanting to talk at once. Dad took me off for a cup of coffee at a nearby café on our own, while the rest of the clan went home to prepare a party in my honour.

As we drank our coffee and enjoyed freshly baked hot scones with cream and jam being my favourite treat, we both felt awkward after so long and wanted so much to say, but unsure how to say it. Finally, Dad leaned towards me, pointing his finger in his usual matter-of-fact way.

"You fought in the wrong country, son."

"What do you mean, Dad?" I looked at him in surprise.

"The Commos are here. The country's lousy with them. Damn protesters against the war are making big inroads into government thinking. And they're all communists, the whole damn lot of them."

He leaned back and sighed uncomfortably.

"The support for the war is draining away. What you boys did up there in Vietnam was great for world freedom. I'm so proud of you, son."

Such words I had been begging from him all my life, but right then, they fell on a different and an uncomfortable place in me. He continued:

"But you need to get back here with your machine-guns and clean up the bloody Reds in our own backyard."

"Dad, please don't … go on …"

"Son, I didn't mean to get into politics as soon as you stepped off the train. I just want you to know how proud I am of what you've done."

I changed the subject. "How's Beatie? She wasn't at the train station." Beatie was Dad's second wife. "Is she okay?"

"Well, she hasn't been the best lately, but she's at home looking forward to seeing you. It's good to have you home, son."

I looked at my father and realised where many of my prejudices had come from. Over the next twenty years, both our views changed along with the world. But, right then, despite his fixed opinions, I felt so much love for him.

"It's good to be home, Dad."

21

A RUSSIAN ADVENTURE

In the twenty-four years following my combat tour, I experienced many radical changes in my life. The most significant was probably that I gave up my need to regard each potential female partner as a substitute mother. Second, I looked closely at my self-esteem, which, for some unexplained reason, took a huge dive after Vietnam. I was no longer the self-assured man I was when in the army. My sense of self-worth was replaced with a more cautious approach to life, some self-doubt, with a sparkle of humility and compassion. This was probably the result of being more in touch with my feelings. Fortunately, my lifelong curiosity and willingness to try new things remained with me.

Hence, I embarked on a career of public speaking as a seminar leader, Breath Integration being my passion. This was my new name for my breath-work process, inspired me to travel around New Zealand delivering talks and seminars. Eventually I got invited by interested groups to Australia, America, and Europe.

This confronted my feelings of self-worth and enhanced much of my healing from the war. A big discovery was the fear of standing in front of an audience, which I found more terrifying than going into combat. When I researched the fight/flight/freeze syndrome and why public speaking was so frightening, I discovered a fear of being judged, rejected, losing control and emotionally exposed. This emotional exposure was more threatening than physical exposure for most people. I eventually ran courses on public speaking to overcome one's stage fright, as the term was known by.

I worked with a small group of Vietnam veterans in Australia with resounding success. But most veterans I approached were not interested, many being in denial that anything was emotionally unstable with them, the same attitude I'd had for 15 years after my tour.

I had loved passionately all the women I'd spent time with, but for the first time, I was enjoying being on my own. Kathryn was now living in America and kept in close contact with me. We also shared David, who lived with me for a time when I wasn't travelling. I also stayed in close contact with my two girls, Bernadette and Angela.

On July 7, 1992, I left New Zealand for Russia, where I had been invited by the Academy of Science to run a training course for therapists and aspiring practitioners in Breath Integration.

Russia was going through enormous changes since the fall of the Soviet Union and was nearly bankrupt from the rapid changes that it was not coping with very well. It had been arranged that I would give my services for free, as a contribution to an emerging democratic nation in need of help from the West.

Prior to this trip, I had conducted an advanced Breath Integration training course in England, which had been successful.

Two days before I was to leave for Moscow, I had an intense Breath Integration session with one of my senior students, Eva, from Denmark. I woke up that morning with a throbbing headache, mild diarrhoea and my stomach feeling in knots.

"I think you need a session, Colin," Eva said, as I came down for breakfast, her sharp eyes and intuition missing nothing.

"No. I'll be okay in a few hours." My reply did not fool her.

"I've known you long enough to know when you are avoiding something important. Come on, I'll give you a session."

During the next two hours, I exploded with anger and then cried like a wounded baby, digging deeply into my subconscious and discovering emotions and memories long forgotten. In the end, it got released (integrated) and I felt the joy and the profound relaxation that follows a major integration of buried subconscious fear. The healing I received related to the battles during the Tet Offensive when I had dysentery. The training course, even though I was conducting it, had reactivated that memory both mentally and physically, from all those years before. My healing was a wonderful preparation for my forthcoming trip to Moscow. I was looking forward to a pleasurable anticipation, for I had long since given up my anti-Soviet/ Communist feelings. In fact, I wasn't anti anything anymore, but was open to discover whether I still subconsciously harboured any ill-feelings for a former enemy.

Flying from London, via Copenhagen, I had the pleasure of sitting beside a young Russian woman who was returning home after living in America for twelve months as an exchange student. Our conversation was an interesting and useful introduction to my coming visit.

For some weeks, I'd had a strong feeling that this trip to Russia would be significant. Familiar with premonitions, but this was different. This time it was as though something wonderful, perhaps a great learning, was going to happen.

Moscow airport in 1992, unlike today, had long queues of travellers waiting to have their papers and passports checked. My companion, having recently experienced the American passport control system, had a different reaction, and became quite angry about Russian inefficiency. I suggested she relax and enjoy her homecoming, but I couldn't shake her out of her cynical resentment.

I was met by my host, Sasha, who made me feel very welcome. His English was reasonable, which was fortunate, as I knew only five Russian words. During our drive to his apartment through the middle of Moscow, I had an opportunity to see some of the city. Overall, it appeared drab, unclean, with nothing freshly painted. However, the area surrounding Red Square, which I later explored on foot, was much cleaner, with astounding architecture.

Sasha's wife, who spoke no English, at once made me feel like one of the family, and became my first teacher of the Russian language.

Every day was an adventure for me. Other than Southeast Asia, I had never experienced a culture so foreign. The second day, after sightseeing with Sasha, he had to run an errand and put me on a bus to get home. It was very crowded, and standing in the aisle, a tyre burst with a loud explosion, close to where I was standing. For an instant, I was back in Vietnam. I immediately dived to the floor among the legs of standing passengers, waiting for the second shot, which I instantly assumed to have come from a Viet Cong RPG rocket launcher. Simultaneously, I looked down at myself to see if I was still in one piece and relieved to find that I was. I looked at the man sitting in the seat closest to the explosion, expecting to see him covered in blood. To my surprise, he wasn't, but was dazed. It was then that I discovered the tyre had burst with such force that it had blown away half of the panelling on the poorly maintained bus. We all climbed off, some snickered at my unusual reaction as they looked at me. No one was hurt, but I felt embarrassed, not being able to control my instant reaction to danger. There was still a part of me that triggered my combat mode after all this time.

After that episode, I travelled mostly by taxi with a group of new Russian friends, introduced to me by Sasha. They were always concerned that I was being robbed by paying such high prices for a taxi. 400 roubles were far too much, they would insist. This was because they were only earning an average of 4000 roubles per month. For me, however, a taxi fare was only the equivalent of $2.00, very much cheaper than I would pay back home. At that time, the Russian Rouble was going crazy with runaway inflation at about 2% per day. I would tell my friends to relax and enjoy the trip of an unaccustomed taxi ride. Most Russians used the underground railway (Metro) system, which was more than impressive.

The first four days were devoted to sightseeing, and on the third day, the Director of the Institute, supplied a car. An interpreter also joined us, and as her English was only fair, it gave me a chance to practice my slowly growing Russian vocabulary. The four of us had a wonderful time laughing and sharing feelings and experiences that went beyond words. I could feel the first stirring of a great love for Russia and its people, a feeling that was to grow deep by the time I left two weeks later.

It was strange for me that almost every street we drove down had been partly dug up for repairs, though there were no workmen present. It seemed that, at the end of winter, the minister for public works would draw up a list of all the roads that needed repairing, and then order them all to be dug up in readiness for the repairs. The repair work would start on only one or two roads at a time, regardless that the rest of Moscow resembled a bombed site. Pedestrians were accustomed to scramble uncomplaining over the piles of rubble and broken concrete whilst negotiating the non-existent footpaths.

My sightseeing was well planned by my new Russian friends to the many historical sites around Moscow. My guides took me to the Kremlin, Red Square and to many cathedrals, which were being restored after seventy years of closure under Communist rule.

Early one afternoon, we had some difficulty finding a cafe for some food and refreshments. After a long search, we finally found a small cafe with only two items on the menu: some sort of grain pancake and Pepsi Cola. I saw high on a shelf some pure apple juice imported from Poland, for which, to the horror of my friends, I was happy to pay eighty-five roubles. The meal for four of us, including the juice, cost me only 285 roubles, along with some head shaking at me being 'ripped off.' It charmed me at their desire to protect me from what they regarded as unscrupulous merchants.

After having travelled for some considerable time around Moscow, I gradually became aware that I had seen only two shops. Whereas, the footpaths were lined with street hawkers, usually older women, selling anything from one packet of cigarettes to many baskets of fruit and vegetables.

Wanting to see more than street markets, I eventually asked my guides if I could visit a typical Russian shopping centre. At first, they were reluctant, but I persisted, and they finally relented. We entered a rather drab building which gave little sign that it contained shops at all, being more familiar to the over-advertising of shops in the West. I think they thought that the western advertising culture was more attractive. We were at once confronted with large queues of people waiting to be served. We stood in line for over half an hour, eventually to arrive at a counter where the shop assistants were especially unenthusiastic, to the point of open rudeness. Service simply did not exist. The merchandise I looked at was very inexpensive, though the quality was poor. I bought a scarf, as I had been feeling a chill from the wind and was aware that the summer weather can be very changeable in Russia.

The next day, I met with the Director of The Academy of Science, my sponsor, his assistant, and a training team of five people who would assist me over the next eight days. Only one of them could speak English that was only marginally better than my Russian. Fortunately, we had an interpreter for the meeting.

I briefed them all on my requirements and they were more than helpful. We discovered at that point that the information handouts on which I based the course had not yet been translated into Russian, even though I had sent them ahead some months before. Though the handouts ran to over fifty pages, the person responsible assured us they would all be ready and printed by the next day, in time for the beginning of the course.

We arrived the next morning at a school that was being totally redecorated, reminding me of the Russian road repair system. Every room and corridor were in shambles, with only one gang working in one room. Throughout the entire school, there was only one toilet in working order.

Thirty-one students, together with my training team, were assembled in the school hall. The information handouts had not arrived, nor had an interpreter. After an hour of panic, and reorganisation of as much as I could of the lesson, the interpreter arrived who knew nothing of the subject I was to talk about. Our first session was gruelling, and it took five hours to cover what I would normally cover in one. The interpreter did his best, but many students were having difficulty in understanding what I was talking about. This stressful situation was relieved through the help of a young psychology student from Lithuania. She spoke good English, and she often had to correct my interpreter in his terminology, but it was still painfully slow and frustrating for everyone.

Despite the total organisational chaos, the hearts of these Russian people were open, understanding and patient and this made the whole process work, much to my surprise. The next day, some information handouts arrived, and they had found a new interpreter who understood a little more about the process I was teaching. By this stage, I had surrendered to the situation and my anxiety levels found some breathing space. After rearranging my program notes, the course flowed with more ease. Using the early chaotic situation as an example of dealing with stress, having just battled with my own, resulted in a clearer explanation of how Breath Integration worked. This was to my teaching advantage better than I had hoped. My new translator, Larissa, was one of the students, and she was excellent, even though she had not been trained as an interpreter.

During the breaks, I spent time with Olga, the young psychology student from Lithuania. She was delightful and; her being glad of the opportunity to speak to someone in English; I invited her out for a meal the following evening.

We planned to dine at a large hotel near Red Square, but had some difficulty getting in, despite the restaurant being almost empty. We were finally successful when Olga suggested I give the doorman a bribe, which was the normal way to get things done in 1992 Moscow. She nodded when I showed her 600 rubles as being enough, and then handed it over and was ushered into a waiting room, much to my amusement. Even then, the waiter kept us waiting for twenty minutes for a table, a sign that perhaps my bribe should have been higher. It was obvious that he was trying to show who was in control, and my companion became embarrassed and resentful that, as a foreigner, I should be treated in this way. After we had finally been seated, we were presented with a menu with nearly fifty items to choose from. When we came to order, however, we found that only two items on the entire menu were available – salad and sausage! The meal was basic, but surprisingly tasteful; the service was non-existent. Despite this, we spent a delightful evening discussing where Russia was at that point in history, split between the ending of the Soviet Union and a new beginning of capitalism. Most young Russians, like Olga, were hopeful of a better life under a new system of government. I was unsure that they would repeat the mistakes of the West, such as runaway consumerism, corruption, manipulative advertising, and the emotional dependency on consumer products. Despite the depth of our discussion, we could keep it light and entertaining.

I had been single for nearly two years after my breakup with Kathryn. Olga was young, beautiful, and I felt my attraction to her when she gave me a subtle hint that she was available. Not understanding such a different culture and her being my student, I thought it prudent not to go down that avenue.

Olga helped me in finding my way home via the Metro. I was truly impressed and delighted to see several underground stations that were elaborately decorated with symbols and portraits of Russian heroes, both of the Communist revolution and of the great patriotic war and victory over Nazi Germany. The carriages were clean, though spartan, with a noticeable and refreshing absence of graffiti. Being sensitive to my feelings and energy I felt a sense of safety in Moscow, quite in contrast to New York, which I had visited the year before.

Four days into the course, I noticed that about 80% of the class were totally committed to the lessons I was presenting. The rest were quite the opposite. Some would fall asleep; others would return late from breaks and were occasionally disruptive. I found this to be a challenge. Fortunately, many of the lessons were experiential for the participants, so that gave me a break from lecturing. It was also interesting to note that despite these people having lived under the restrictions of communism for over seventy years, there seemed to be a very subtle, and probably unconscious, desire to resist, rebel and even sabotage whatever was being presented. It was common to find many of the assignments designed to get people in touch with their feelings and thought-provoking exercises were sometimes deliberately done incorrectly. I suspect this was an example of the independent streak that had survived in a recent past controlling regime in such a tenacious people.

The lunch break was interesting and spent mostly outside in the summer sun. We had each brought food for a shared meal. Many of the participants would hand me small cakes, or tiny, delicately prepared sandwiches, crammed with a variety of fillings. I would soon have a pile of food in front of me that was more than I could eat. I was touched by their hospitality and generosity. We would all talk and laugh our way through the meal, and though I seldom knew exactly what they were saying, I understood the conversation flow, often helped by sign language. The flow of warmth made me feel both humble and exalted that we could share so much together with very few words.

One lunchtime, halfway through the training, a Russian woman appeared at my side and informed me in excellent English that she was there to teach me the language. So, each lunchtime for 30 minutes, she tutored me on basic words and simple phrases, but more on the alphabet of the Russian field of language. Initially, I could not speak much better, but I began to understand the written language, to read signposts, to connect short sentences and, importantly, to understand more of how Russians think. It is true that a language is so much connected to the culture. Inna was a wonderful teacher for that short period each day. I had always doubted my ability to learn a foreign language, but now, for the first time, I began to think that it would be possible.

On the fifth day of the course, a student about my age stood up and spoke through my interpreter.

"I have been doing breathwork and rebirthing for two years and came to this training more out of curiosity than to learn a new science. I realise now that it's no coincidence that I have come here, because Colin was in Vietnam. So was I in Vietnam as an instructor for the Viet Cong. I saw action against the Americans at the same time Colin was there."

I was stunned. Suddenly, I was looking at someone who was my former enemy. Feelings about the war welled up, and it was several minutes before I could speak. There was neither hostility nor warmth that flowed between us, only our own personal memories. Everyone in the room felt the energy between us as we looked at each other from across the room. Neither of us knew what to do with our feelings that were arising, but mercifully, someone rescued the situation by asking a question about an aspect of breathing and its relationship to mental health, and the lesson continued.

Later in the afternoon, the ex-Russian soldier/instructor had a Breath Integration session that brought up painful memories from twenty-four years earlier. As he battled with such memories, he exploded angrily, then cried like a hurt child for nearly half an hour. I knew exactly what he was going through, having had a similar session only a week earlier in England. Gathering myself, I went over and sat beside him. Then, after a time, when I felt our energies were aligned, I wrapped him in my arms. Then, holding him like a baby, I gently rocked him, feeling the pain slowly leave his body. Many of the students in the class broke down and openly wept at seeing two former enemies now united in loving friendship. I was unaware of the commotion in the room, being fully involved with a man whom I could never again hate, for whom I could only feel love for. It was a moving experience for everyone, but more so for me and my new Russian brother.

Afterwards, my new friend hugged me and openly wept with joy. Then, looking straight at me, he spoke in a torrent of Russian, too fast for me to understand a single word or even for my interpreter to translate. It was unnecessary. His message was obvious.

At the end of the day's session, over a coffee, surrounded by much of the class, I tried to find out from him what part of South Vietnam he had been operating in. I found out that he was there during the Tet Offensive. But the commotion of so many people looking on, also wanting to speak their excitement at our common experience, that was all I could find out. I understood through the translator him saying that we may even have traded bullets at each other. He finished saying that he was leaving the course as he had found what he had come for: a major healing from the war. The last few minutes before we both left for the day were the most precious. Without a word being spoken, tears in our eyes, we looked deeply into each other's heart and felt a huge weight being lifted from both of us and replaced with a deep brotherly love. Then, with no ceremony, he turned and walked away. I will remember this precious moment to the end of my life.

I now knew why I came to Russia.

23

THE PRECIOUS GEM I STOLE FROM RUSSIA

That night, while walking towards the Metro on our way home, our group stumbled into a Communist rally. Waving their red and hammer and sickle flags, they were mostly old men and women protesting about the rapid changes taking place in their country. The lack of future job security and the dangers of widespread unemployment under the new democratic government fuelled their protest. There was a lot of argument and finger-pointing between them and bystanders. A great deal of fear and anger could be seen in their faces as they protested the uncertainty of the new politics in Russia. Committed as I am to democracy, my heart went out to those disorientated people in a swiftly transforming political situation.

Alcoholism was a real problem in Moscow. It was a common sight to see men lying unconscious in the street, clutching an almost empty bottle of some spirit. With each passing day, I could feel more of Russia's pain, as my love for this country and its people grew.

Every lunchtime, I found myself sitting next to a young woman who was having quite an effect on me. Each of the students moved me, but there was something about this woman that fascinated me. Her name was Marina. She had a degree in Russian literature and language and was a writer for a theatre company. She had studied English, but never practised until now, which made her speak it a little better than my Russian, but despite this, we communicated very well. It was wonderful to realize that there are many forms of communication other than words. We shared a meal together one evening after class, and a mutual feeling of attraction began to grow. She was 32, attractive, and had an excellent sense of humour. For the rest of the course, I was very aware of her presence in the room.

On the second to last day of the training, one of my assistants suggested I should be more authoritative and insist that everyone return promptly to the class from their meal breaks.

"They are used to being more directed. You have to be firmer with these people," she insisted.

"Maybe they do have something more important to discover here," I replied. So, after the next break I addressed the whole class:

"It has been suggested that I become firmer regarding starting times, returning from breaks, completing group and partner discussions and processes, to ensure that you all get the most out of this training." I paused to gauge the reaction before continuing.

"However, I have no intention of doing this. I want you to understand that you are fully responsible for your part in what happens here. You will get out of this exactly what you put into it. If you choose to waste your time by coming late, refusing to do the discussion processes, and not taking the full advantage of what the course offers, then it's your loss. If this applies to you, then perhaps you need to look closer at your own motivation for being here and take responsibility for your own process. But I will demand nothing from you, nor will I take responsibility for your decisions. Does what I'm saying make any sense to you?"

There were many nods around the room, and I felt an immediate response from almost everyone present. Afterwards, I reflected that it might have been beneficial to have given that speech a few days earlier.

The last day brought about the delivery of the rest of the information handouts. At this stage, I couldn't use them, but not having all the handouts much earlier was no longer an issue for me. I'd long since become content with the course to unfold as it was.

After a moving closing ceremony during which each student connected with each other at a heart level, the class put on a concert in my honour. I was more than happy that Marina sat beside me. We spoke little, but a beautiful energy flowed between us, and we found that we often glanced at each other. At one point, I briefly touched her shoulder to highlight something I was saying, and I noticed she leaned in towards me in a receptive response.

The concert included many singing traditional folk songs, others danced, and it was a beautiful display of Russian culture. In one humorous presentation, six students acted out a group Breath Integration session and did everything opposite to the lessons in the course, making it totally hilarious, which brought many laughs from everyone. At their conclusion, I announced how delighted I was that they had learned the process so well. Then, several announced they would like to sing to me in English, but as they couldn't speak the language, they jokingly said that they would dance for me in '*English*'. They performed a beautiful Russian folk dance. I later commented on how beautiful they did it in '*English* ', but I noticed that the dance had a strong *'Russian accent.'*

At the end, they all thanked and showered me with gifts and compliments, and then warmly hugged me before I left. It was touching to know that I had a caring Russian family that goes beyond words.

The next day was for sightseeing and a group of us and, much to my joy, Marina also joined us. We travelled out of Moscow to an old monastery that had also once been an ancient fort. On the way, our driver asked me what I thought of the roads, which were so bad in this part of Moscow, that he was forced to drive much of the way on the opposite side of the road and often on the footpath to avoid the numerous and deep potholes. I laughed and answered that I found them interesting. Then Marina smiled, and in her broken English added.

"I know this story. During second World War, as Russian forces were falling back everywhere, they were evacuating all that they could carry, factories, quickly harvested crops, contents from houses and deserted shops. German advance was slowed down because of the bad state of the roads. One German officer said that, in the Russian urge to evacuate everything, they had also evacuated the roads!" We all laughed, and I was impressed at her sense of humour.

The two days before I left Moscow, Marina took time from her job and agreed to spend the remaining time with me at my request. They truly were magical, and I could feel a love not only for Russia but also for her growing in me. By this stage, her English had improved through the short time we had spent together. Her earlier studies in English and her practise with me had improved the communication between us.

To help my Russian pronunciation, she got me to practice sounding out each street sign we came to. We made a game out of it with a point system and had so much fun. She had the same type of sense of humour I had and announced with a straight face.

"I have special powers and can grant the ownership of any building in Russia. For every street name you pronounce nearly correctly. I will grant you the ownership of any building of your choice, beginning with the Kremlin or Red Square if you want it. But you must for, for ..."

"Forfeit?" I jumped in.

"Ah, yes, forfeit any if you get one wrong."

Walking down many streets, parks, and other places of interest, enjoying the game and being very conscious of each other made it a perfect day.

Then we came across a 'STOP' sign written in English. I looked at it, twisted my head to look at it from another angle, and shook my head. "Nyet" (no), I don't know how to say this one." I looked at it upside down, sideways, close up and said, "Oh dear, I don't understand this at all. I'm going to have to lose one of my buildings. You're going to have to help me with this one," all the time rubbing my head and face in mock bewilderment.

She laughed and took me in her arms, exclaiming in English, "You are such a large boy!" We looked into each other's eyes and laughed together. I told her that in my country I would be called a 'big kid'! We laughed again, then stopped and held each other's gaze. Of all the treasures I had found in this amazing country, I knew that I'd found the most precious gem a person can find.

On my return to the United States a taxi driver, after learning of my visit to Russia, told me he knew of some people in Congress and in the U.S. military who would love to destroy the Ex-Soviet Union now that it is weak. I felt sick to my stomach on hearing that. I can only trust that wisdom will prevail both in Russia and in the West, and that all the former hostility between East and West will be finally healed.

On August 28, 1992, I returned to Russia and was with Marina for two weeks. By this time, I was sure that I wanted her as a partner. In October, I returned to New Zealand after completing my world lecture tour via Australia, where I started writing this book. On arriving home, I made arrangements for Marina to come to New Zealand. Meeting up again with Kathryn and David, who had come from America for a visit; she was delighted that I had found happiness again.

In November 1992, Marina arrived at Auckland airport into my waiting arms. My writing of the first edition of *Wounded Warriors* was well on the way by her arrival, with some unwelcome side effects.

Through November and December, Marina and I set up house together, amid my relapses into emotional pain as I explored through my old Vietnam diaries that rekindled terrible memories. This must have put a doubt in her mind to question her decision to have come across to the other side of the world to be with someone who was loving in one moment to suddenly become an emotional wreck in the next. But she understood I was going through a powerful healing period and was totally supportive in my process.

Near the end of the diary, dated April 26th, 1968, was a blank page with just the date and nothing more. I remembered deliberately leaving the page blank to show my loss of memory at the time. My only recollection was watching the rainwater trickling down the tent ropes two days after the supposed event. I knew something significant, probably terrible, had happened, but my mind refused to allow any memory to recall it. As I sat at my desk, I could feel a strong, uncomfortable feeling welling up in me, like a panic attack. I looked up from my writing the moment Marina walked into the room. Taking one look at me told her I was distressed.

"Come, my darling, and lie down with me. You need to breathe and connect with the pain that is coming up in you, right now."

Shaking my head and feeling the fear, knowing that it would be so easy to push it down again and not have to deal with whatever was coming up. The energy was similar to the session I had in England several months earlier, but even stronger. This made me more afraid to face whatever was coming up.

"No, I'm okay," I lamely said.

Taking me by the hand, she guided me to our bed and before I could settle myself to prepare for the Breath Integration session, my mind became flooded with the memory of the dream of being shot through the face and killed. It was one of the most powerful sessions I had ever had, as I relived the fear of dying in the most grotesque and horrible way. More astounding was the intense physical pain in my stomach where, in the dream, two bullets had found their mark. At the worst moment of the session, for some minutes, I felt this amazing phantom pain. I could feel Marina's energy reaching out to me, embracing me with her love. About 20 minutes of breathing, being present with my feelings and my resistance to feeling them, eventually the storm of fear was released. As my body relaxed through the integration, the gentle memory of water gently trickling down a rope coupled with the intense pleasure of joy that often goes with the release of a major fear pattern.

It has always interested me how the mind blanks out traumatic memories as a way to emotionally survive. When the trauma is reactivated as part of the healing process, or when an event triggers the trauma, the memory returns. This is one of the main reasons why many traumatized people avoid connecting with painful memories and discussing their feelings about it. Yet, this is the most direct way of healing the trauma.

When healing is completed, which is the release of the suppressed fear, the memory is vividly remembered, but without the pain. It is just an event with the wisdom of what we learn from it.

Yet, the resurfacing of the trauma of my phantom death, followed by the integration and release that happened back in Vietnam, the memory remained hidden until this session with Marina, 24 years later. This shows that there is still much we don't know about intense trauma in the subconscious mind.

I wondered, more out of curiosity than dread, how much longer I am to experience these powerful healing sessions. For some months, now I'd had quite a few. Yet, the fear of the session was disappearing and replaced with a new level of acceptance that made each session an exhilarating experience. In time I was to understand that trauma and suppressed feelings form a husk around us like skins of an onion. As the healing begins, and as each layer is released, the layer beneath suddenly becomes exposed and sensitive, ready to be released. Once the healing is started, it progressively gets easier. I could readily see profound changes happening in me, resulting in being more sensitive and emotional on one side, and being more loving, happy, but more importantly, a feeling of inner freedom was making itself known. This new freedom was not being controlled by earlier destructive beliefs and urges. This was such an encouragement to keep going, no matter how long it would take. Permanent progress was revealing itself.

Afterwards, as I lay in Marina's arms, feeling my joy and her love, a wonderful thought struck me.

"You know what?"

"I feel a great desire to go back to Vietnam and bury some ghosts. Will you come with me?"

"Of course, I will come with you. But is it really that you want to bury some ghosts, which is what you have been doing for the last 24 years."

"Ah, yes, a poor choice of words, but it is probably a Freudian slip as a part of me still wants to bury, um … bury my feelings. I think going back there will help release a lot of traumas for me."

24
RETURNING TO VIETNAM

Marina and I arrived at Ho Chi Minh City (formerly Saigon) airport in the late afternoon. It was January 28, 1993, exactly twenty-five years since the start of the Tet offensive. What caught my eye first was the oval shaped concrete hangers scattered around the airport that once housed the American fighter bombers during the war. The hangers stood there deserted and overgrown with vegetation, a stark reminder of the painful past.

We were greeted at immigration and customs by stern-faced officials in the uniforms and badges of my former enemies. I felt nervous waiting in line, hoping they wouldn't search my bags and discover my combat uniform. I had brought it with me to be left in Vietnam, together with any pain that I still carried in my body and mind. Had we been searched; this would have been difficult to explain. The man in front of me had his bag searched, which increased my anxiety. Then, on my turn, I moved to the counter, smiling at the customs officer with all the charm I could muster. He looked back at me unsmiling, hesitatingly, as if undecided. I suppressed any body language signals that might give my nervousness away and imagined that he was my loving brother to help in my deception. He looked at our bags, then back at me and waved us through. I looked back at Marina, who was following, and winked at her with a sigh of relief.

At the next counter, which was immigration, we were thoroughly questioned why we had come to Vietnam, and I insisted we were only there for a holiday. Before we left New Zealand, our travel agent had advised me against revealing that I had fought in the Vietnam war. At the end of the war, all Allied soldiers had been convicted in the Vietnamese highest court and ruled as war criminals to be arrested and imprisoned if caught. Vietnam had just overturned this law, and some veterans had returned to the country with no problems. But I felt it better not to mention my war service to save any complications.

On clearing immigration, our taxi took us to the Norfolk Hotel in Ho Chi Minh City, where we received excellent service. At breakfast the next morning, Marina spoke to me gently.

"Remember, you have returned to Vietnam not as a defeated enemy, but as a mutual victor with the Vietnamese people. Look at how these waiters are treating us. You've come here as their friend to enjoy your shared victory from the war." I looked at her lovingly and relished in what she said.

Later that morning, we walked around the local area. The roads were bustling with an endless stream of bicycles and Honda motor scooters, so crossing to the other side was done with some difficulty. The streets were dirty, noisy, busy, and lined with shops and street vendors selling a wide variety of products. In the side streets and alleys, people lived out their whole lives, it seemed, on the pavement. Here they cooked, ate, played with their children, urinated, and washed their clothes.

We went for a ride on a trishaw, a bicycle with a seat in the front for two passengers. As we travelled about taking in the sights, there were many ex-US service military vehicles where the American white star had been crudely painted over. Most of these vehicles discharged clouds of black smoke from neglect and badly tuned engines, leaving our throats coated from their emissions. I was captivated by the different smells that greeted us every few metres, and the exotic sights at every turn. It was how Malaysia and Singapore were twenty-five years ago, before they gained the sophistication and trappings of the late 20th century. The barricades and barbed wire defences around prominent buildings were still in place eighteen years after the war had finished in 1975. What struck me most was a sense of an American presence that still lingered after all this time. At any moment, I expected to see an American military police jeep, or trucks filled with US marines, or American GIs walk past.

I found myself often breathing deeply as my emotions were stirred from half-forgotten memories, mingled with some anger. From the window of our hotel room that looked out on the street below, I would stand watching the passing traffic and hordes of people. I found it impossible to simply be here now and was constantly drawn back to painful events of 25 years earlier. Whenever I saw Vietnamese males around my age or older, I wondering on what side they had been on, VC or ARVN?

Suddenly firecrackers began sounding off in the street below as part of the Tet holiday celebration. The staccato explosions sounded like gunfire, and I felt quite sick. I imagined bodies lying in the street after a gun battle, a common occurrence during the war. The latent violence within me surfaced again, and I doubted the decision to have come back to Vietnam.

Later that afternoon, we visited a museum which depicted Vietnamese political and military history from 1930 to 1975. Each large room was devoted to a specific period, with the first covering the misdeeds of the French colonial rule. The second hall presented the Japanese occupation and their oppression of the Vietnamese people during the Second World War. The third hall covered the atrocities and defeat of the South Vietnamese government and, of course, the 'American imperialist invaders'. Ho Chi Minh featured prominently in each hall together with other Vietnamese heroes from the period on display. At the entrance of each hall, we were met by a charming young woman dressed in traditional Vietnamese costume who escorted us around, explaining carefully in poor English, about each photograph and exhibit. In the hall that covered the most recent war, the woman, on learning that I was from New Zealand, pointed proudly to a photograph which showed a New Zealander in Hanoi protesting against the Allies during the war.

"New Zealander very good." She smiled at me, and I returned her smile, marvelling at her innocence of the hatred that fuelled that era.

"American people very good. American military very bad," she parroted, as the routine narrative was obviously well rehearsed. Then I saw a faded photograph of New Zealand infantry lined up on parade at Nui Dat, shown by the black sweat scarf that only New Zealand combat troops wore. I looked closer, careful not to appear too interested, to see whether I could recognise anyone. The photograph was too faded to identify anyone, but I thought I recognised several guys from Five platoon. With insufficient time to take a closer look, I couldn't be sure.

On the 31st of January was Marina's birthday. We both woke up in a slightly depressed mood, a state of mind which steadily got worse as the day progressed. I needed to be on my own and went for a walk. I took a trishaw to another museum with a provoking title: War Crimes of Aggression in Vietnam. It was mostly dedicated to atrocities committed by the Americans. There was a strong emphasis on the My Lai massacre when about 500 unarmed South Vietnamese civilians were killed by US troops in March 1968. Other photographs and exhibits showed B52 airstrikes and the spraying of 75 million litres of Agent Orange, the lethal defoliant chemical dispersed over much of South Vietnam. There were many photographs of foetus malformation and deformities in babies, and many others that showed Americans torturing and killing VC and innocent Vietnamese people. As I stood there looking at the hideous exhibits, I realised that the existence of such a museum is a sign that the world, including the Vietnamese people, still has a great deal of anger to release. There was no mention, of course, of the many atrocities committed by the Viet Cong and the torture and execution of thousands of village leaders, often in front of their families. Whilst I was not surprised by the lack of impartiality, I found it sad that the Vietnamese government does not acknowledge that atrocities can be and always are committed by both sides in any war. War, after all, is an atrocity, for expecting and indeed, demanding young men and women to kill their brethren who think differently. To fight for your country is a politician's polite way of saying to kill for your country. And killing destroys the very foundation of the survivor's psyche and creates a generation of wounded warriors.

I left the museum feeling sick.

My driver suggested in broken English that I might like to see the old American Embassy, abandoned in 1975. I walked in the now deserted and overgrown grounds of what was once the representation of the American presence in Vietnam. It was a large, architecturally Western designed building, surrounded by a high concrete wall. As I walked around, I realised that exactly twenty-five years to the day, to this very hour, was the scene of heavy fighting, as US marines and military police fought to defend the embassy from the attacking VC on that fateful day of January 31, 1968. I remembered the film clips I'd seen soon after the event of this place, in which the frightened voice of a young Marine guard was recorded and played on the TV news.

"Oh God, they're coming. Please help us!" was all that was heard. Then silence. They found his body and the other Americans who had died that day when the embassy was retaken a week later.

Suddenly, stopping to walk, I heard a faint sound of men yelling excitedly as in the heat of battle. I looked towards the main gate from where the sound seemed to have come from. Nothing, just the usual passing traffic. 10 minutes later, I heard the yelling again, this time from the south wall, and could have sworn the voices were in English, with the unmistakable American accent. I turned and looked in that direction. Again, nothing. I shook my head to think clearly. Minutes later, I heard a very faint scream of terror, and then it faded away once more. All the voices seemed remote, much like barely hearing the very low volume of a radio or speaker way in the distance or as if in a dream. The hairs on the back of my neck stood up, reacting to what seemed to be happening. Then I heard a distant crackle of gunfire and explosions. I stood, transfixed by phantom impressions. It was as if I had tapped into a time warp and could hear, though faintly, the actual sounds of a quarter of a century earlier at this precise time and place. I couldn't be sure if my mind was playing tricks on me as the effects were so subtle, or whether I had transcended time, enabling me to recapture that precise turbulent moment.

I walked around the grounds and building a second time and then a third and each time in two specific places where I stood very still, I could hear these distant sounds coming to me in waves, only to fade out, as with the tuning down the volume of a radio. Having a vivid imagination, it probably was my own mind playing tricks from this whole setting and my 'jangled' emotional state. Whether it was just my imagination, the experience was distinctly eerie, and I left feeling unsettled.

I returned to the hotel feeling slightly depressed, but a little better than when I'd left several hours earlier. At the reception, I booked a car for the next day, with a driver to take us out into some jungle near Bien Hoa. I wanted to be near the site of the day when we attacked the VC camp in the early hours of the morning of February 1, 1968. This would be the 25th anniversary of that terrible day. I planned to bury my uniform and perform a small closing ceremony to symbolise a Qabalistic healing ritual. That evening we celebrated Marina's birthday, and we both felt in better spirits. The hotel staff had prepared a cake and provided live traditional Vietnamese entertainment, so it was a wonderful evening.

At 8.30 the next morning, our driver arrived. His English was poor, so we had some difficulty explaining what we wanted to do. He drove us to the town of Bien Hoa, where I suggested we visit the old American airbase. I had seen it from the air in 1968 when we flew over it by helicopter to our operational area and was interested to see what was left of it from the ground. After driving around for a short while, our driver got directions from a local and 15 minutes later, we drove into the front entrance of the base. The barbed wire barricades and machine-gun concrete bunkers were still in place, but deserted and overgrown. The faded and rusty sign over the gate was in Vietnamese.

The driver pulled up beside a more recently built shed, got out of the car, and went inside. Minutes later, he reappeared, followed by a stern-faced Vietnamese military officer in his mid-thirties. I knew we were in trouble the moment I saw him. Through the open car window, he spoke rapidly to us in Vietnamese, and then switched to Russian. On hearing this, Marina opened the car door and jumped out, speaking to him in her mother tongue. The rapid conversation was impossible to follow, and I cursed I had not been more attentive in the Russian lessons Marina had been giving me in New Zealand. The officer was aggressive in both speech, manner, and body language, demanding to know what we were doing here and what we wanted. I realized this was now a Vietnamese military base, and that I had put us in grave danger by insisting on coming there. I heard Marina explain that, as we were celebrating our birthdays, we were looking for some jungle to have a picnic. As proof, she reached into the car and grabbed her passport and pointed to her date of birth. Still, the officer was unconvinced. She reached into the cab and grabbed the birthday cake given to us by the catering staff the night before to show the officer. For the first time, he slightly smiled and relaxed, charmed by Marina's disposition. He spoke rapidly to our driver, giving him instructions of some kind. Then, returning to Marina, he explained he had trained as an officer in Russia for a time and could speak some of the language. A few minutes later, we were on our way again.

"His Russian was not too good, but I think he understood what we wanted," Marina said.

To be certain, I asked our driver if he understood that we now wished to find some jungle. He nodded but drove back to Ben Hoa village. On arriving, he drove slowly past shops, appearing to be looking for something in particular.

"Do you understand that we now want to find some jungle, nothing in town?" I asked again. He just nodded, but kept driving slowly, continuing to look at the shops as we drove past.

"Cake," the driver finally said. "You need cake."

"No, we don't want a cake. We already have one." As I gestured towards the cake on the seat. Then pulling out the tourist Vietnamese phrase book and finding the word jungle, showed it to him and pointing to the word and a photo of native jungle, saying.

"We just want to find some trees and jungle. Do you understand?" Finally, he understood and at last turned the car around, heading out of the town and hopefully towards some jungle. Marina and I smiled at each other as we realised what instructions the officer had given to our driver.

We drove for twenty minutes finding no jungle. There were paddy fields and rubber trees, but no jungle to be found. Clearly, in this part of South Vietnam, the Americans had destroyed it all with Agent Orange. 'That, I must agree, was one of their atrocities,' I grimly thought.

We finally decided to stop inside a rubber plantation. After getting out of the car with my uniform, diaries and combat boots carefully wrapped up in brown paper and coloured plastic bags, we looked around for a likely spot to perform the ritual I had in mind.

I wanted to do my brief ceremony as close to the battle on this day, 25 years earlier as possible. To give me my bearings, I asked our driver what way was north. As he didn't understand, I pulled out my old military map of this area of the original battle site to show him I wanted to find north. His eyes widened, and he shook his head to show that he was confused and distressed about me showing him what he must have recognised as a military map. In my effort to get the information I wanted; I did not realise the danger I was putting us in. He must have concluded us as spies, by first wanting to see a Vietnamese military base and then flashing a military map. I felt myself getting annoyed at having a driver with such little understanding of English. My frustration was aggravated by Marina's insistence on me putting the map away, her recognising the danger, and urging us to move at once deeper into the plantation. I finally relented, and we instructed the driver to return in an hour.

Then we started walking further into the plantation of rubber trees, hoping to find a likely spot.

"It is important that I find north, to pinpoint the actual location of our battle." I complained as we walked.

"Perhaps so, but you don't seem to realise that our driver could be working for the Vietnamese intelligence service, or the equivalent of the KGB. It's strange that our driver knows so much about us. He obviously told the military officer that I'm Russian. Our driver is probably very suspicious of us. And now, you showing him a military map. I'm feeling very uneasy about all this."

"Oh, my gosh, you're right," I breathed deeply to let go of my irritation that had turned to concern.

"I also feel that we could be in some trouble from my foolishness. Let's find a place quickly and get this uniform and diaries buried before we are caught with them."

Minutes later, we saw our car disappear out of sight towards Bien Hoa. We looked at each other in dismay. Marina's forehead showed worry lines. I'd learned that her intuition was always right, so there was no time to waste.

"Come on, this spot will have to do," I pointed towards a clearing between the rows of trees. I pulled out my small, fold-up shovel and a candle. Placing the candle in position, I lit it, together with some incense, then dug a small hole beside where I was sitting. We stayed seated and innocently appearing, as local plantation workers walked by without them paying much attention to us. I didn't want to attract any attention, but so far, I had done my best to advertise to the world the very opposite. Then a convoy of what appeared to be military trucks passed by on a road 100 metres away. The trucks were filled with men in white uniforms and my uneasiness increased. I had Vivid images of spending the rest of our lives in a Vietnamese prison on charges of espionage.

I took several breaths to calm myself to prepare for my simple ceremony. After several minutes of gathering myself, I unwrapped my uniform. Picking up the trousers, I refolded them and carefully placed them into the hole. Then, likewise, with the shirt. Both items of clothing were well-worn from extensive wear and were faded from having been in storage for so long. Next, the combat boots. Their soles had been worn down from months of patrolling in the jungle not too far away from this spot. The boots were followed by my black scarf/ sweat band, with its little white kiwi emblem. Then the dog tags that we also wore around the neck for identification and to show our blood group. I found it hard to drop these last two items into the hole, feeling a strong attachment to them. My jungle hat followed. It had holes in it from the sharp bamboo I had encountered during one of our patrols. I smiled as I remembered once kidding to my young daughters that the holes were from VC bullets. Each article I handled gently and respectfully. My previous despise of the past had largely gone and replaced with a gentle reverence. Now, however, I felt I was ready to close this chapter in my life forever.

The last items were my three diaries, written in small notebooks, now falling apart through age. I picked up the middle one with a large '2' on the cover, opened it, found the page dated February 1, 1968, and read aloud:

"It's my birthday, but it's gone unnoticed as I have other things on my mind, like staying alive. We were woken at 0500 to prepare for the attack on the VC camp. My guts are in a terrible state, constantly rumbling, and I'm having to relieve myself every ten minutes or so. I barely slept a wink last night. Will I be alive tonight to complete this day's entry?"

I sat there, memories racing through my mind, and I read on.

"The firepower from the airstrikes and artillery fire was overwhelming on the hill just above us, as we moved up in preparation for the coming battle ..."

A later entry... "Only two VC bodies were recovered from the battle.

They'd taken their dead and wounded with them as usual …" "Des Hirini was killed today from a contact. I feel so terrible, I could just die!"

As the memories overwhelmed me, I burst out crying. From the years of sessions, it was now easy to let my feelings express themselves in this very healthy way.

I felt Marina sit behind and snuggled into my back with her loving support. That brought up a confused mixture of love and horror at the same time. Such a concoction of mixed feelings sent my emotions into greater turmoil of feeling out of control. I first resisted, then became fully present with them, and they released.

Over the next 15 minutes and after several more emotional waves, it finally completed itself as I felt that incredible relaxation and joyful feeling, as usual, after an integration. I also felt grateful for Marina's presence, which greatly helped the feelings to come up and be released. Minutes later, I nodded, that I felt okay, and Marina moved away to give me space.

I dried my eyes, read some more, and ten minutes later closed the diary. Then, placing all three in the brown paper bag, dropped them into the hole, with this dedication:

"I place into the soil of mother earth these objects and symbols of pain, grief and horror, which I now choose to no longer resist, but allow to be a part of my life experience that has taught me so much. And if I do resist any feelings from the war, which is probably likely, I commit to being as fully present with this resistance as much as I am able to." This removed any pressure of having to do it right in the future. Michael Freedman's words came to me. "There is no 'right or wrong' way to do it. Either you do it or not, and either way will be right for that moment." I continued.

"Should any pain and fear linger here, I ask that it be taken to a place of presence for healing. I acknowledge the fear and shame I have held for the things I had done against the young men and women I'd met in battle. May their pain be released with mine."

It was on the tip of my tongue to add that I was deeply sorry for my actions, but there was no sign of the feelings of guilt that I had carried for 25 years. It seemed that this session minutes earlier had released this and replaced with a new level of innocence that was beautiful and unfamiliar.

As I whispered these last words, my heart opened to release another dam of tears, but these were tears of overwhelming joy.

"Today, I'm not 47, but only one day old as I begin my life anew. As a Vietnam veteran, I have often looked to use my war experiences to excuse and justify my uncaring and angry behaviour towards those who loved me.

Also, my limited thinking that I am a victim to other people and situations. Now realizing that all difficult situations were from my own making, coming from my own unconscious. I am ready to take responsibility for how I think, feel, and behave. I am now willing to release all my blame and excuses for being a damaged veteran from the war."

I suddenly sensed a wall of resistance to this idea. I smiled compassionately to myself, as I grieved for the potential loss of my security blanket of excuses and status as a wounded warrior. The question that I'd lived with for so long could I cope without my excuses, justifications and instead being my real self, and all that it entailed? To be powerful and vulnerable, sensitive, and yet open? I sat still as this new idea and feeling flowed through me, letting it fill me.

"I commit to being a peaceful emotional warrior. I will face my resistance towards my feelings as a peaceful warrior!"

Taking a deep breath, I moved forward and filled in the hole in case I was tempted to change my mind and fall back into being a victim again. Then I sat there again without moving, soaking up all these new feelings and thoughts to course through my body and mind. As I did so, a new thought came to me:

'Everyone acts for the highest good, for the wellbeing of all people. Beneath the selfishness, the greed and the fear, beat a noble heart of courage, love, and integrity in everyone of us. Within each person is the spark of divine perfection. We just have to let it shine through.' This thought was strong as I remembered the noble deeds of those young men who fought for what they believed in, on both sides, in these jungles that were once here. The thought deepened. 'Even those acts of atrocities that were performed were done from perhaps misguided minds who deep down felt victimized and, on the surface, believed that their actions were for the common good. For me to judge their actions is to live in ignorance of my suppressed fear and my own unconscious fear-driven agenda.' This last thought was like a completion. We smiled at each other.

I looked up and saw our driver 100 metres away, watching us through the trees. I placed some leaves over the filled in hole, not to be discovered, blew out the candle and extinguished the smouldering incense. Marina took me into her arms.

"Congratulations, conquering hero. Congratulations, my peaceful, emotional warrior," she said, and her eyes were filled with love and admiration. We gathered up our belongings and, arm-in-arm, walked back to the waiting car.

I knew I had much more healing still to do over the coming years. But I was feeling good about my emotional state as it now was. As I thought about the fear of dying in battle and being shot through the face was no longer there. I recognised the fear of feeling my own fear (resistance) was my greatest challenge. Yet there was the comfort, and a willingness to do this. I was no longer afraid to face the future emotional storms. Apart from feeling love, joy and inner freedom, the healing itself had been an enormous journey of self-discovery, making the whole process worthwhile.

This simple ceremony had shown me that most people carrying trauma were most afraid, not of the situation that caused the trauma, but having to face their own feelings about that trauma. Even though my recent sessions have been pointing this out to me, right now it has never been clearer for me.

Three hours later, back in our room having a cup of tea, we still had a feeling of potential danger, perhaps of an ongoing investigation of us being spies. Then, suddenly, something energetically changed. We both felt it together. I looked at Marina.

"I've a feeling that the Vietnamese Intelligence has just finished investigating us and have concluded that we are not spies."

Marina nodded in agreement and smiled. "Yes, I feel much better now, too." I don't know how we somehow knew that a danger had suddenly passed.

"I can understand why they may have been suspicious of us," I continued. "You're Russian, and my passport shows I travel often, particularly to America. Then we wanted to find some jungle near a military base. On top of all that, I started pulling out a military map!" I laughed as I thought about it. "Our poor driver must have been beside himself at our behaviour, which wasn't exactly normal, was it?"

"I was trying to warn you." She smiled, shaking her head.

The next morning, I slipped out of bed early and looked out of the window at the street below. I saw the scene was unchanged, yet in every way it was totally different. People still rode by on their scooters and bicycles, and the noise and bustle were the same. Then I realised that the only thing that was different was me. The American presence that was so strong yesterday was gone. I was no longer looking at Saigon of 1968, but at Ho Chi Minh City in 1993. Firecrackers suddenly erupted a street away as part of the continuing holiday celebration. But they were only firecrackers. Emotion welled up inside me, and a tear spilled onto my cheek. A tear of joy in that I was only one day old and enjoying the celebration of life.

Thoughts of the war were still there, but the dread I'd lived with for 25 years was gone.

I crawled back into bed beside Marina and whispered into her ear my favourite Russian phrase. "Ya Lublu Tebya. (I love you). I love all the Vietnamese, all the Americans and all the Russians. They're all wonderful. I feel so much gratitude for all that has happened in my life, especially for the healing from war. Thankyou Mr Gurdjieff and Michael Freedman for teaching me to be more aware and to reach out for my higher self."

"You know Colin," Marina answered as she stretched and yawned. "It's no accident that Mr Gurdjieff, one of your most important teachers, was a Russian."

"By goodness, you're right." I could now see how all events are interwoven, and marvelled that Marina, a Russian, and a so-called former enemy, was now united with me in love.

We spent the rest of the day sight-seeing, eating exotic foods, sharing laughter and joy. On our way to the airport the next day, our taxi driver, who could speak good English, was very friendly and talkative.

"I was an officer in the South Vietnamese Air Force during the war. I worked with many Americans. They okay." I asked.

"Did you meet any New Zealanders during the war?"

"Oh yes, and Australians as well. New Zealanders and Australians very good, very funny with their jokes."

He evaded my questions about how he was treated by the Communists after the war. He told us, however, that he had undergone three years' corrective training, and had then worked for the government for ten years for meagre wages. Only in the last few years had he earned a basic wage by driving a taxi. Marina squeezed my hand when she sensed I was about to launch into a discussion about my previous visit to Vietnam. I took the hint, kept quiet, and sat back to enjoy the leisurely drive to Ho Chi Minh Airport. How different I felt and indeed, how different I was from the last time I left Vietnam.

25
FINAL WORDS

A year later, in a meeting with Michael Freedman, finally cleared up the question of the altered state of consciousness, when everything had slowed down as in slow motion during my most desperate moments in combat.

Michael was a psychologist, who had graduated with honours years before I met him in 1978. He had combined his unorthodox psychological approach with mysticism* giving his work an interesting and greater potency. He insisted that no real healing can happen without including emotions in the healing process. This influenced my coming years of research and development of Breath Integration. When I asked him about my weird experiences, he replied in this way:

"I have never experienced war but expanded consciousness would explain it this way. That elevated level of awareness of complete presence is a powerful and incredible experience that rarely happens in a person's life.

There are two ways to reach expanded consciousness. One is through unconditional love of another person. This is generally not available to the average person, because we all love with an ulterior motive. To get loved back, or for sex or any number of hidden agendas that we consciously and unconsciously search for from another person. The second is through intense fear. This is readily available to every person, because we all have fears. When a person makes their fear fully conscious, and faces it head on,

* Mysticism: Mysticism has nothing to do with black magic that some religious groups believe. Michael's mystical approach focused on expansion of awareness leading to deeper spiritual experience.

even gives up all hope of survival they start to enter the timeless present moment to such a degree that consciousness suddenly expands, and they witness reality quite beyond ordinary awareness. Your explanation of your weird experience, Colin sounds like that is what happened to you. Let me explain it this way.

Imagine a cup is falling off a table. In normal consciousness, the person's mind would register the cup just leaving the table. Then another frame of experience when the cup is halfway to the floor, then another frame when the cup hits the floor and shatters. When a person enters the present moment with one's whole being, awareness expands. The mind captures many more frames of experience in a single event compared with normal consciousness.

For example, the mind first registers the cup beginning to fall. Then another frame of experience close to the first and then another close to the second, and so on. During the cup falling, the mind would capture many more frames, giving the slow-motion movie effect you spoke of. It's not that time has slowed down; it just means that you capture more frames of experience of the same event and in the same time span. Because you are fully present with everything happening inside yourself as well as outside. This would connect you with your true self, which only knows love, deep happiness, and inner freedom. You are totally at peace and your body is totally relaxed. In fact, you have become one with all life, and that is why you had difficulty being a soldier at such times."

"So, what about guys who experienced euphoria during battle but are still physically stressed?" I asked.

"Such an experience was because of the person's frozen state. They would probably see only about one or two frames of experience from the falling cup. The euphoria is a coping skill for overcompensating the feelings of intense fear in the frozen state. Probably, most men in battle would close down and feel nothing. The euphoria only occasionally happens. This is probably what your army doctor diagnosed your experience to be, not knowing anything about the healing properties of the present moment."

Because most people are more afraid of their own fears than actual dangerous situations are why this experience is so rare. They just fall into one of the fear responses, the fight/flight/freeze syndrome and consciousness is reduced rather than expanded.

I further asked.

"So, expanded awareness is about living life to the full?"

"Yes. This is the true meaning of that expression. Most People think living life to the full is about entertainment, many sexual experiences and partying. It's really about living life to the full in the present moment, and that could include the sheer joy of simply washing the dishes in the state of presence."

I couldn't stop myself and further asked.

"So, what I experience was expanded awareness?" Michael nodded, and I continued.

"So does that mean that a person experiencing expanded awareness might be slightly more conscious, perhaps more spiritual, than the average person?" He looked hard at me and then, after a long pause, said.

"No. not at all. It just means that everything was lined up for a person to have such an experience as you did. You tapped into a psychic muscle by accident and not by design. We can only measure true spirituality not in how many spiritual muscles you have, but in how much unconditional love and inner freedom one experiences. Not as a belief, or as a philosophy, but as a way of living one's life to the full. Having fewer beliefs that one is controlled by is also a good sign of true spirituality. And that you asked this last question shows you are still seeking my approval and praise for your experience. Does that sound right to you, Colin?"

"Oh, yes, I think I still have a long way to go."

"Yes, I think so, too. But you have made a good start."

That was my last conversation with Michael and was probably one of the most important lessons I ever received from him in the 17 years of knowing and working with him. A few months later, I was saddened by his death. I have deeply missed him ever since, but he left his inspiration with me that has carried me through the deepest of healings and exploration of my work.

During the final stages of this book, has revealed some important insights for me. It was the healing itself, which was the greatest benefit I received from this entire experience. The feelings of love, happiness and inner freedom have been amazing, but were only the effect. It was the release from trauma that was even more amazing as it gave me a small glimpse of my true self and the unfathomable and limitless power, we all possess inside. Without being traumatized in the first place, I would not have had all these amazing experiences of healing. That is why I said at the beginning of this book, Vietnam was such a gift for me. Without those dreadfully painful experiences, I would have lived an ordinary life and be denied the greatest journey: 'The journey from my head to my heart.'

Most of us have been traumatized throughout our lives and carry the status of the wounded warrior, feeling victimized by our personal Vietnam inside. We live in fear that the worst events that have happened may happen again. But it is not possible, for subconsciously, we have a built-in survival mechanism connected to our fight/flight/freeze syndrome to ensure that our worst traumas are never repeated. But the fear will remain until we release it when it is met by becoming fully present with it.

May I be bold enough to say that the trauma of our personal painful experience is a blessing, for it gives us the opportunity to go inside and discover our courage, inner strength, and find the integrity of who we really are.

If we understand this, the way clears for true healing. If we can embrace the past hurts with gratitude for the lessons learned and experiences gained to make us more loving and joyful, then we will have found freedom.

I salute the peaceful, emotional warrior in each of us!

Of the millions of young men and women who fought in this nightmare, each has their own story to tell.

This was mine – Thank you for walking with me for a while and allowing me to share my thoughts.

COLIN P. SISSON.

Tae noa Ki te huihuinga ano

Until we meet again.

POSTSCRIPT

Those that are interested in finding out more of the healing process, Integrative Presence, can order my recently published title: "The Truth of Your Moment." This describes the complete process in an easy-to-follow text. Order from: colinsissom.com

and soon to be created web site: www.integrativepresence.com

Or purchase directly from Amazon, search: The Truth of Your Moment, by Colin P Sisson.

A special message to Vietnam veterans and their families.

The jungle warfare training we received actually trained us to suppress our feelings that caused so much trauma.

One of the most serious causes of trauma amongst our combat troops was in the very army training itself. In Malaysia, doing our jungle warfare preparation, much of it was centred around the drill for contact with the enemy - 'contact front,' 'contact rear' and 'contact left or right.' The drill was activated whenever any member of a patrol, mostly our scouts, saw the enemy, was to open fire and the man closest to him would yell, 'Contact front!' With that, every man in the patrol would run forward towards the sound of battle, then spread out, offering a wide front facing the enemy with the maximum firepower to win the firefight.

Other times, when the lead scout saw an enemy in the distance, would send back the silent thumbs down signal, indicating a firefight was imminent. The whole patrol would go into the drill of a contact front, by moving forward silently until the scout or the enemy opened fire.

We practised these drills hundreds of times in the jungles of Malaysia until we got it down to clockwork precision. However, during actual combat operations in Vietnam, with every contact, our training was that when each ran forward, while his mind was sending the signal of danger to the rest of his body. If the mental/emotional/physical response was anger, then it would cause no trauma, being part of the 'fight' reaction (as part of the fight/flight/freeze syndrome, the natural fear response). But for most men, the first 3 or 4 enemy contacts felt enormous fear, the flight or escape part of the syndrome. To run towards danger when fearful is against every instinctual mental/physical system inside of us and the only way to cope is by suppressing the fight/flight/freeze syndrome and one's feelings all together. This was hugely damaging psychologically. By about the fourth or fifth enemy contact, anger began to take over from the fear, but this was more the result of suppressing previous fears than being a natural response. By now, as veterans, we thought that we had become battle hardened, but in most cases, we were just more suppressed than guys going into battle for the first time. This showed up through serious PTSD later in life when old, suppressed fears re-surfaced, often activated by then current difficulties, such as in health, relationship, or careers.

Dealing with the combat stress was much harder for the married guys as they had more to live for. Us single men still went through the suppressing cycle, but not as severe as the married guys. This concludes for me that no married man should ever have to go into combat. ***And no single man should ever have to go either!***

The waiting for something to happen was nearly as traumatic as the actual combat

An overlooked cause of trauma was in waiting for something to happen. Those endless days of patrolling and hours lying motionless in an ambush site, or on sentry was mind-numbing, with the prominent thought: 'What if...' When an enemy contact was made, the first feeling was often 'relief,' and then the fear response would kick in. I was fortunate that I never got lost in worrying about meeting the enemy. But those who did were, in fact, reliving an imaginary conflict inside themselves repeatedly, and it drove some men crazy.

Many veterans I've met in recent years have often made similar discoveries that I have written here.

Those of you that are still struggling with health, relationship, or financial issues could be still unconsciously fighting the inner conflict. I invite you to read 'The Truth of Your Moment' and come home to all that you are: a true hero in the act of defending your country. Now it's time to take care of yourself.

ABOUT THE AUTHOR

Colin Sisson was born in Levin, New Zealand in 1946. In 1965, at nineteen, he joined the army in a youthful, patriotic urge to serve his country. Having passed the difficult selection course, he trained with the Special Air Service (SAS). Later, he transferred to the Infantry, where he was posted to the 1st Battalion RNZIR (Royal New Zealand Infantry Regiment stationed in Malaysia. After 12 months of jungle warfare training, he was selected for V2 Company, the second New Zealand infantry company to tour Vietnam.

He crammed in a lifetime of experience in 6 months, but he met the downside of humanity in its basic urge for survival that is found in any extreme situation. Despite the anguish and the agony that is found in men who face life and death situations daily, there was a positive experience to be found, the incredible journey of self-discovery.

On returning to New Zealand, mentally and emotionally exhausted, he took an interest in psychology to start the search for himself, having glimpsed it through the terrors of combat. In 1980, he was introduced to the Qabalah and breathing techniques, which was to transform his life. Over the following years, Colin discovered that the healing of emotional trauma itself was the gift of self-discovery and became a successful seminar leader to pass on his discoveries. The founder of Breath Integration and co-founder of Integrative Presence led him to write ten books, to express his insights. He is internationally known as a speaker and writer in the United States, Poland, Russia, Britain, New Zealand, and Australia.

A recipient of the Queen's Commendation for Brave Conduct, a civilian award, for rescuing a woman trapped in a blazing vehicle after a motor accident. Colin continues to learn and share his knowledge with others through his writings on healing and personal development.

Marina Kitchatova

V2 COMPANY NOMINAL ROLL

Attached to V2 Company from 161 Artillery battery.

Casualties: KIA Killed in action.

WIA Wounded in action requiring Hospitalisation. A further 35 men were wounded in action but remained on duty after medical treatment.

Rank	**Name**	**Given Names**	**Casualties**
Major	Worsnop	Brian Thomas (Company Commander)	
Capt	Dudman	Michael John (2nd in Command)	
W02	Faulkner	David William (Company Sergeant Major)	
LCpl	Allan	David Stuart	
Pte	Allen	Rosswold	
Pte	Apiti	Ronald Mihi	
Pte	Avery	Leon Terrance	
Pte	Awatere	W. R.	KIA in W Company
Cpl	Bassett	Michael John	WIA
LCpl	Beckham	Ray Harold	
Pte	Berridge	W.C.	
Pte	Booker	Norman James	
Pte	Boyce	Ian Charles	
Pte	Bray	Frank James	
Cpl	Bristowe	Hukarere Mamaeroa	WIA
Pte	Brown	Terrence Murray	
Pte	Burgering	Colin Richard	
Pte	Card	William Bennett	
Pte	Charman	Leonard James	
Pte	Claude	Peter John	
LCpl	Collins	Albert	WIA
Pte	Cornes	William Edward Morrin	
Pte	Cowie	(Andy) Andrew Panton	
Pte	Cummins	Howard James	
Pte	Curtis	Joseph Thomas	
Pte	Dallow	John Redwood	
Pte	Dargaville	Richard (Dick)	
Pte	Dempsey	Selwyn Keith	WIA
	Doak	Dennis Walter	
LCpl	Douglas	Malcolm Murray	
Pte	Draper	Gerald Wallis	WIA

Rank	Name	Given Names	Casualties
Pte	Duggan	Brendan Vincent	
Pte	Duncan	Graeme James	WIA
Pte	Easton	Richard John	
Gnr	Ellwood	Stuart (attached from 161)	KIA
Pte	Eriwata	Russel Te Pononga	
Sgt	Ferguson	Lyall James	
Pte	Flower	Rodney Charles James	
Pte	Framhiem	William Taerikimataki	
Pte	Gaunt	George	
Pte	Gardner	John Ralph	
Pte	Gawler	Robert Maxwell	
Cpl	Girling	George Fredderick	
Pte	Godsiff	David Wilson	
Pte	Gordon	John Nesham	
LCpl	Grace	Stanley Sydney George	
Pte	Greenhough	John Cedric	
Pte	Griffin	Dennis Alvin	
Cpl	Hanna	William James	
Pte	Hapuku	Robert Te Raingiutu	
Pte	Harmer	Edwin James R	
Pte	Hatu	Te Miro Oraukawa	
Pte	Haua	Allen George David	WIA
LCpl	Haworth	Rodger Barrington	
WO2	Hayward	Willian David Anthony	
Dvr	Heather	Meau Nicholas	WIA
Pte	Hema	Dick Henare	
Pte	Henry	George Albert	
Pte	Heremaia	Michael	
Sgt	Hill	Gregory James	
Cpl	Hill	Robert Stanley	
Pte	Hirini	Haere Desmond	KIA
Pte	Hoani	(Joe) Joseph	
LCpl	Hori	Arthur	
Lt	Howell	Anthony Gordon	
Pte	Hunt	Gary Patrick James	
Cfn	Hunter	Brian Joseph	
Cpl	Hunter	Paul Paora	WIA
Pte	Hunter	Tuakau	WIA

Rank	Name	Given Names	Casualties
Cpl	Hurliman	Joseph Robert	
Pte	James	Robert Gary	
Pte	Johnson	Desmond George	
Cpl	Kelly	William Richard	
Pte	Kinane	John Alfred	
Cpl	King	Gary Graeme	WIA
LCpl	Kingi	David Karepa Pukeho	
Pte	Komene	Hini	
Pte	Lambert	John Robert	
Pte	Leat	Gilbert Nickie	WIA
Pte	Levy	Bruce William	
Pte	Linley	John Herbert	
Pte	McCormick	Kenneth	
Pte	McGee	Joseph Edward	
Pte	McKean	Patrick Henry	
LCpl	McLachlan	Anthony Fraser	
Pte	McPhail	Daniel James	
Pte	Mackey	Hamana Waaka	
Pte	Martin	John Ihaia	
Pte	Matene	Hohipa	
Pte	Mathews	Rex Jan	
Sgt	Mato	Whakaro Rangi	
Pte	Mills	Garrie James	
Pte	Mitchell	(Mitch) Vian Christopher	
Pte	Monk	John Fredrick	
Lt	Mountfort	Richard Murray	
LCpl	Murphy	Brian Laurence	
Pte	Murray	Kevin Blair	
Pte	Nant	Raymond Hardy	
Pte	Neame	(Blue) Roy Henry	
Pte	Niwa	Ross Patrick Rangi	WIA
LCpl	O'Connor	Brian Daniel	
Pte	Ormond	Kemp Tamuia	
Cpl	Paipa	(Buck) Wiremu Te Parkarotorangi	
Pte	Panther	Bruce	
Pte	Parkes	Arthur Clarence	
Pte	Paterson	(I.B.) Ian Bruce	
Pte	Peddie	Graham John	

Rank	Name	Given Names	Casualties
LCpl	Peni	Lewis Ruatiki	
LCpl	Perawiti	Patrick Puke	
LCpl	Perkins	Peter Innes	WIA
Pte	Pewhairangi	Charles	
Cpl	Phillips	Louis Ruihana	
Pte	Pleydell	Roger Gordon Walter	WIA
Pte	Poa	Cecil Edward	
Pte	Pourewa	Karanga	
Pte	Presnall	Ronald Graham	
Pte	Pringle	Anthony David	
Pte	Pritchard	Ronald James	
Cpl	Puia	Albert Sydney	
LCpl	Rameka	William Bert	
Pte	Ratima	Desmond	WIA
Pte	Rawiri	(Toy) David	
Pte	Richards	Eric John	
Pte	Rickard	Colin Ivan	
Pte	Riddle	Colin Bruce	
Cpl	Runga	Joseph Te Okoro	
Pte	Ripikoi	M.W.	
Pte	Ruru	Potatutahu Bill	
Pte	Sadlier	Harry	
LCpl	Sandford	Denis Steward	
Pte	Shale	Michael Richard	
Lt	Shattky	Derek Graye	
Cpl	Shaw	Roy Colin	
LCpl	Shatford	Morris	
Pte	Simeon	Samuel Joseph	
Pte	Simmons	Brian Thomas	
LCpl	Simpson	Gary	
Pte	Sisson	Colin Purvis	
Pte	Simms	Graham John	
Pte	Smith	Albert Francis	
Pte	Speight	Howard Cecil	
SSgt	Steele	Gerald Turkington	
Pte	Sturmey	Edward Koro Jewal	
Pte	Taare	(BB)Whare Mira	
Pte	Tahana	Kereti	

Rank	Name	Given Names	Casualties
Pte	Tauhinu	(Grease Gun) Jock	
Cpl	Taukamo	Tai Te Ngahere Oriwa	
Sgt	Tataurangi	Edward	
Pte	Tautau	Barney Te Whanauapani	
Pte	Tawhara	John Robert Sydney	WIA
Pte	Thompson	Clive Anthony	
Pte	Te Rangi	William Aniheta	
Pte	Timu	Edward Tumanako	
Pte	Te Ua	Walter Horton	
Pte	Tocher	James Conway	
Pte	Toohill	Barry (attached from 161)	
Pte	Tuhoro	Peter	
Cpl	Vautier	Walter Stephen	
Pte	Waaka	David Rawiri Paora	
LCpl	Watson	Douglas	
Pte	Wealleans	Douglas Wayne	
LCpl	Wharewera	Jake Hakota	
Cpl	Whitaker	Thomas Douglas	
Pte	White	Kani	WIA
LCpl	Whittaker	Malcolm Grant	WIA
Sgt	Whitworth	John Russell	
Sgt	Williams	Robert George	
Cpl	Wilson	Howard Owen	WIA
Lt.	Wilson	John Gilbert Hamish	
LCpl	Wiringi	Ginny Andrew	

More books written by Colin P Sisson

REBIRTHING MADE EASY – 1985. (Out of print)
A gateway to Self-Knowledge, Aliveness and Compassion

YOUR RIGHT TO RICHES – 1986
A practical guide to creating wealth and fulfilling your dreams.

BREATH OF LIFE – 1989 (Out of print)
Experience happiness, love and peace through Breath Integration.

WINGED THOUGHTS FROM THE HEART – 1990
A selection of beautiful thoughts written in prose of a life's journey.

WOUNDED WARRIORS – 1993 (2nd Edition 2021)
The author's experience in Vietnam and the discovery of himself.

INNER ADVENTURES – 1998
The journey Home, back to our hearts, back to who we really are.
The more in-depth presentation of Breath Integration.

THE NEXT STEP – 1999
A recommended follow-up on Inner Adventures. A practical in-depth exploration of awareness through love, joy and inner freedom.

SECRET OF THE TWELVE STONES – 2010
A novel based on a true story of a man who goes in search of buried treasure in the Amazon jungles, where he finds the treasure within.

INSPIRED LEADERSHIP – 2021
The effective management of self, and the people we lead through the heart, the head and super consciousness.

THE TRUTH OF YOUR MOMENT – 2021
The liberating power of breath, presence, and conscious living

Website of Colin: www.colinsisson.com

Made in the USA
Monee, IL
04 November 2026

67375847R00144